Calm Kids

a guide to using natural therapies for children

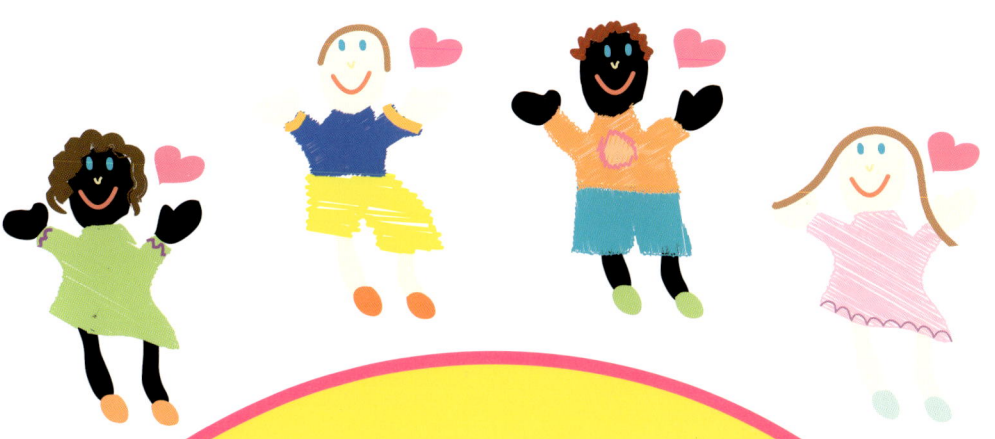

Dedication

To the children I have connected with throughout my life. The lessons I have learnt through their adventures have taught me more than I have time to share.

I also dedicate this book to all of the people in this world brave enough to take on the parenting role. It is the most important and responsible work to do on this planet. Interestingly, it comes with no directions.

First Edition Published in 2003

Second Edition Published in 2005 by

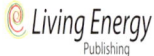 Living Energy
Publishing

Living Energy, Australia
Email: toni@livingenergy.com.au

National Library of Australia cataloguing-in-publication data

Jefferies, Jennifer, 1961

Calm Kids: a guide to using natural therapies with children

2nd Ed.

Includes index.

ISBN 0 9750966 0 5

1. Child development. 2. Aromatherapy. 3. Child psychology.
4. Therapeutics, Physiological. I. Title

305.231

Please Note

The information contained in this book is not intended as medical advice, but as general
information only. The author/publisher cannot accept responsibility for any mishap resulting
from the use of essential oils, or other therapeutic methods described in this book. My advice
to the reader is to realise you are an individual, and as such, I recommend you consult a
professional aromatherapist or healthcare professional if treatment or advice is required.

Edited by Simone Tregeagle, Ink Communications, Sydney

Author Portrait by Kirsten Heritage, Studio Heritage, Townsville

Cover, Layout and additional Drawings by Toni Esser, Living Energy Publishing, Gold Coast

Printed by Everbest Printing Co, China

Jennifer Jefferies

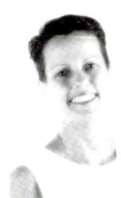

 author

 professional speaker

 health practitioner

Jennifer is a qualified aromatherapist and naturopath but better than that, she's also a real person. She's travelled the road to corporate burnout where she decided to change her life, become a health practitioner and help others to learn what she did about living a life in balance.

Her background includes 14 years as a professional speaker and for the last 22 years she has owned and managed retail stores and natural medicine clinics in Australia.

Today Jennifer speaks to corporations throughout Australia, New Zealand and Southeast Asia. She is a refreshingly down-to-earth, engaging and informative speaker who leaves her audiences feeling empowered about the things they can do to achieve balance in their lives, rather than feeling guilty about what they're not doing!

Jennifer's passion in life is informing people about ways they can integrate natural therapies into their work and personal lives to achieve the feeling of really LIVING and not just EXISTING.

Jennifer's books include:

★ 7 Steps to Sanity
★ Sanity Savers - Tips for Work/Life Balance
★ Amazing Scents - A Guide to Aromatherapy
★ The Aromatherapy Insight Cards for Intuitive Aromatherapy
★ Essential Woman - Guide to Using Aromatherapy for Women
★ If You Want Great Skin...Throw Away Your Cosmetics
★ Network or Perish - Learn the Secrets of Master Networkers

Acknowledgements

This is the second edition of *Calm Kids* and with this edition we chose to have some very special kids illustrate it for us. The kids come from my circle of family and close friends.

I would again like to thank our 'cover girl' Alexandra Reinhardt, gorgeous daughter of our dear friends Michelle and Shane Reinhardt. Since the first edition was published Alex now has a new little sister, Jazzlyn. Both Alex and Jazz have contributed some of their drawings to this edition.

Thank you to my sister Michelle's children Marissa, Emma and David and to my brother Lee's boys, Cameron and Jaiden. Thank you all for your very cool, colorful and inspiring artwork. It is great to have you kids in my life to play with.

To my dear friend Jim Doyle's son Lachlan, thank you also for your wonderful illustrations. Your work inspired us to illustrate this book.

And finally I would like to thank all the kids, big and small that I have connected with and treated in my naturopathic clinic over the years. It is my work with them that inspired me to write this book.

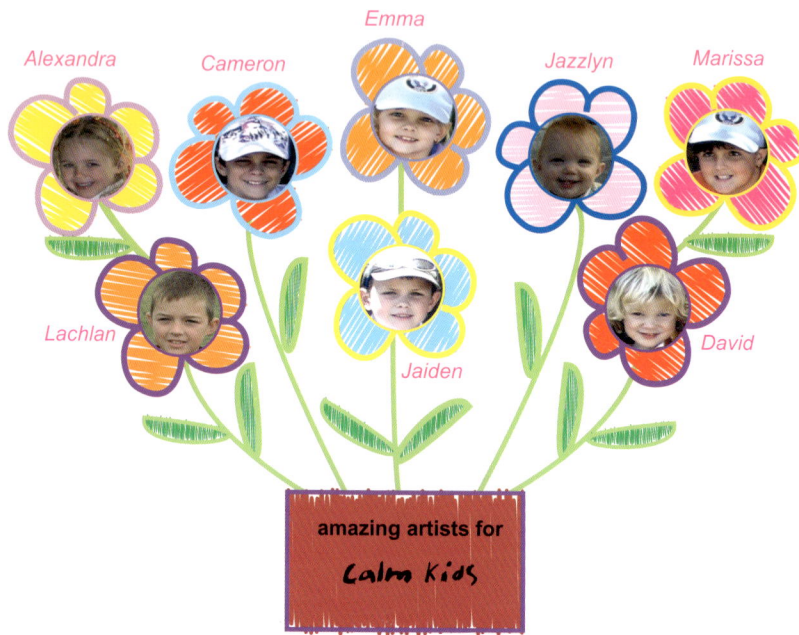

Alexandra   Cameron   Emma   Jazzlyn   Marissa

Lachlan   Jaiden   David

amazing artists for
Calm Kids

Contents

Introduction

In case you hadn't noticed, kids don't come with instruction manuals, and as much as children are just little versions of grown-ups, they are also more complex in some ways and far simpler in others. Children tend to run more acute ailments than chronic, but that doesn't make things any easier; with children there is so much more emotion involved.

As a naturopath and aromatherapist I think I have seen just about every childhood ailment there is. And I've seen how natural therapies, aromatherapy in particular, can help parents and children alike to better deal with some of the many challenges that life throws at us every day.

Throughout fifteen years treating clients in my clinic, I had the pleasure of assisting many people in using natural therapies to go through the process of conception and pregnancy, right through to seeing the new baby born and then grow into a young child. In our retail stores we were constantly confronted by tired and worried parents wondering how they could use natural therapies with their children, and for years I presented a workshop called *Calm Kids*, which is what led to the development of this book as a simple and practical guide for parents in using natural therapies, and particuarly aromatherapy.

Aromatherapy is suitable for children and babies of any age, but it must be used with care. Aromatherapy essential oils are potent natural compounds which must be used according to the directions and advice of a qualified aromatherapy practitioner. If you follow the advice and dilution recommendations in this book, you will be using aromatherapy safely and you will find it an easy and enjoyable form of natural therapy that can bring many benefits into your family's lives.

Alexandra, the little cutie pictured on the cover, is the daughter of our friends Michelle and Shane Reinhardt. They have raised a gorgeous child who has lived with aromatherapy since her birth. Michelle and Shane are aromatherapy consultants who use essential oils and other natural therapies in every day life. And Alexandra just expects that everyone gets to go to sleep smelling the delights of essential oils at night. I remember once when I was working in our retail store, an eight-year-old boy came up to me and told me how he used Lavender essential oil to help him sleep and how if he got a scratch his mum would put a drop of Tea Tree onto the bandage; this type of thing makes me smile on the inside. I remember myself being the 'Queen of bandages' all throughout my childhood. I was a 'go-fast' kid who didn't know how to walk – I raced around constantly and was always hurting something! That is just what kids do and so we have to learn to work with it.

Natural therapies are not new and aromatherapy is not some new 'fandangle' thing for us to play with. All we have done is gone back to the basics, working with nature to treat ailments and to help keep our bodies well rather than waiting to get sick. It's about going back to the times when people had a closer affiliation with nature, and worked with it rather than against it.

Our bodies have been given the power to handle whatever is thrown at them, and kids sure do throw lots of things at themselves. I know through my experience with kids and their parents in my clinic over the years, natural therapies work exceptionally well for both the acute cuts, bumps and fevers as well as the chronic coughs and so on.

Natural therapies are powerful and beneficial in many different areas of life. In this book I have given you some basic principles and methods for integrating natural therapies into your life to help with the many daily excitements that living with children can bring. I have also included recipes that will be useful for some of the bigger kids too, because sometimes teenagers can be even more challenging than younger children.

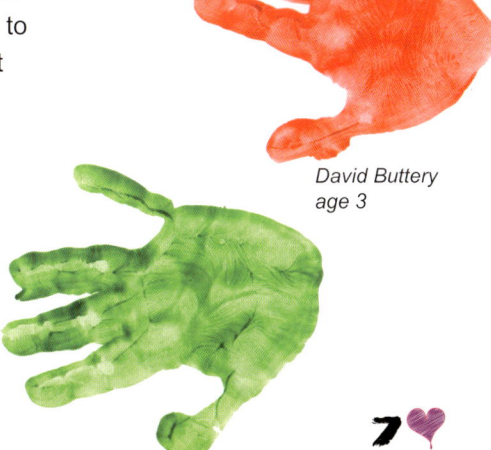

David Buttery age 3

Enjoy the journey!

Jennifer

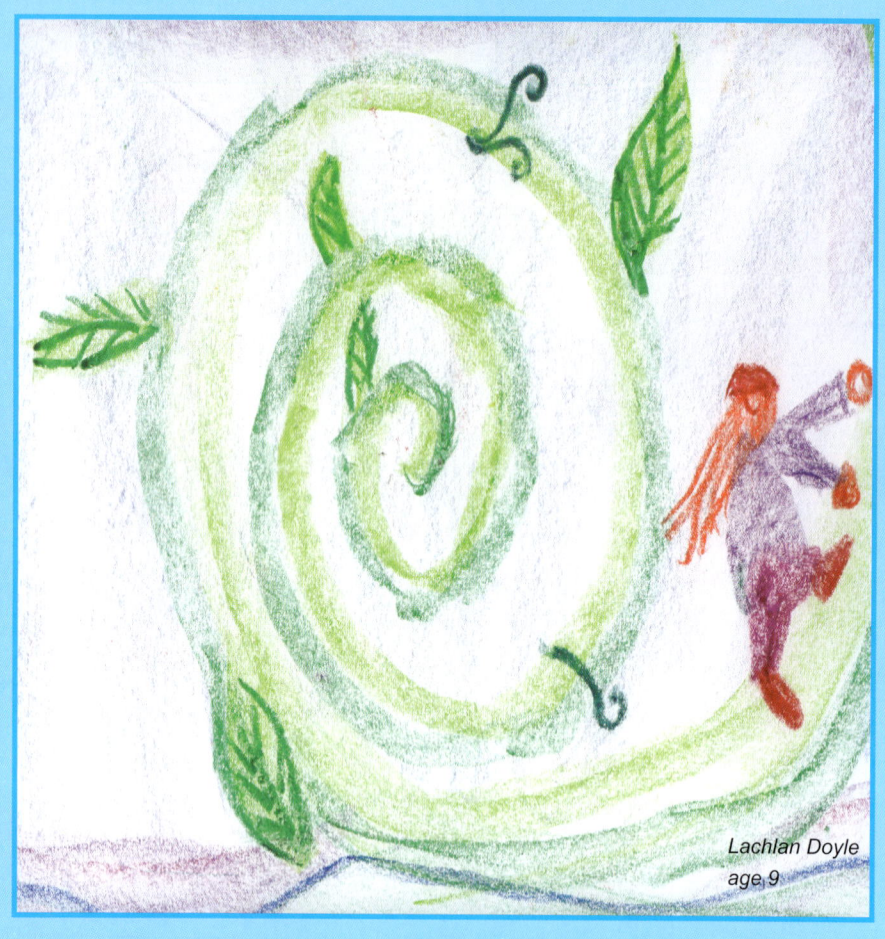

Lachlan Doyle
age 9

⭐ Singing songs at night is a bedtime ritual for our family. **Miss Four** says, "Mum, sing me a song". Mum replies, "I can't think of one off the top of my head at the moment", **Miss Four** says, "Then use the bottom bit of your head! ⭐

Michelle Reinhardt
Melbourne, Victoria

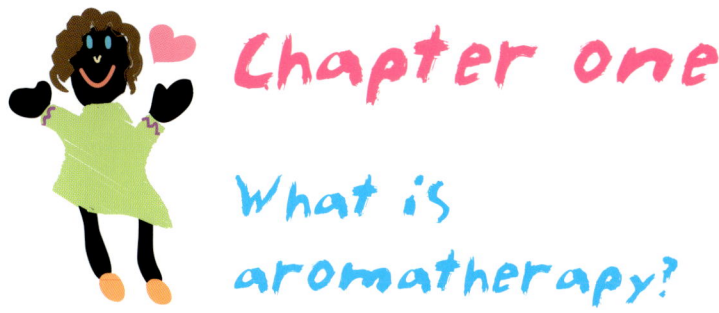

Chapter one

What is aromatherapy?

Aromatherapy is the science of using essential oils for therapeutic, mood enhancing and cosmetic benefits – basically it's old-time pharmacy. Since the beginnings of human civilization, healers have looked to nature to provide remedies. For centuries essential oils have filled dispensaries and provided pharmacists with the raw materials to make medicines. It was not so very long ago that you would take your prescription along to the local pharmacist and he or she would make up your cough mixture or cream from scratch using essential oils and herbs. Today, most of these natural medicines have been replaced with synthetic laboratory-produced drugs. But we are seeing a resurgence in the popularity of natural therapies, and aromatherapy in particular. Women's magazines commonly feature articles about the use of aromatherapy essential oils and specialist aromatherapy products can be found in every department store. Part of the reason for this increase in popularity is because aromatherapy is not only an effective tool for preventative healthcare, it is also incredibly pleasant and very easy to integrate into all areas of life. Because it is so easy to use, people can overlook the fact that aromatherapy essential oils are extremely potent and powerful in therapeutic use and must be used with a measure of care. By following the basic rules outlined in this book, you will learn how to use aromatherapy oils safely and to their greatest advantage. Make sure that you consult a qualified aromatherapy practitioner if you have questions (an appropriately qualified aromatherapy practitioner will be registered with The International Federation of Aromatherapists, (IFA)).

Aromatherapy and wellbeing

Essential oils have many talents, the most obvious and frequently cited is their ability to treat physical ailments such as headaches, aches and pains, coughs and colds, and skin and sleep disorders. Much of the focus in published material and in the work of aromatherapy practitioners is on these physiological benefits of essential oils, and I have also used essential oils to great effect in my clinic over the years with people who want fast relief from physical symptoms. Yet the physical healing qualities are such a small part of the oils' potential. The emotional or subtle side is less well known, yet it can be this which offers the greatest healing benefits. Essential oils can also work on the emotional causes that lead to physical symptoms in the first place. In this book I will refer to both the emotional and physiological uses for essential oils.

So what are essential oils?

Essential oils are the highly-concentrated, aromatic plant essences that can be derived from just about any part of a plant including the flowers, flowering tops, leaves, stalks, fruit rinds, seeds, saps, nuts, bark, roots, resin and berries. The oils give a plant its scent and are essential to its biological processes. In some cases, several different oils can be derived from one plant. The orange tree, for example, gives us Neroli from the flowers, Petitgrain from the leaves and Orange from the fruit. Each of these three oils has its own distinct personality and therapeutic properties.

Holistic aromatherapy recognises that all of the natural and biological components of essential oils work in synergy to produce their therapeutic qualities. Essential oils used in aromatherapy must be 100 per cent 'pure and natural' – meaning that there must be no synthetic materials added to the oil. Most essential oils produced throughout the world today are used by the food flavouring, perfume and pharmaceutical industries. These essential oils are pure and natural, but have also been purified by further distillation and during this process some of the minor chemical constituents are discarded.

The smell of essential oils

Scents can vary in their appeal and effect on different people, depending on the person's individual experiences and chemical make-up. A scent that I adore could be very unpleasant to someone else.

Our memories are strongly anchored to our sense of smell and that can have a significant impact on whether someone finds a particular smell appealing or not. In my teaching I use the example of Lavender. Lavender can be the most relaxing oil in the world, however, if you have a memory associating the smell of Lavender with a distressing experience or person from your past, that memory can be triggered whenever you smell Lavender oil. In this case it would be unlikely that you would receive all of the relaxing benefits of Lavender.

The key to choosing aromatherapy oils is to realise that we are all individuals and that our sense of smell is closely linked to our memories – so choose scents that are appealing to you personally and understand that your choices might be very different to the choices of others.

How do essential oils affect our bodies and minds?

Essential oils are absorbed into the limbic system of the body through the olfactory bulb and cilia in the top of the nose. When you are surrounded by a scent, for example your perfume or cologne, your nose can become saturated to the point where you can no longer consciously smell it. With aromatherapy the same thing happens, but even though you may no longer be consciously aware of the aroma, it is still having an influence on you. When you use your oil vaporiser, for example, after a while you will no longer be consciously aware of the smell unless you leave the room for a while and re-enter. But the oil is still working. People that have lost their sense of smell, or been born without one (anosmia), may be unable to enjoy the aromas but similarly they will still experience the benefits of essential oils as they are absorbed into the body.

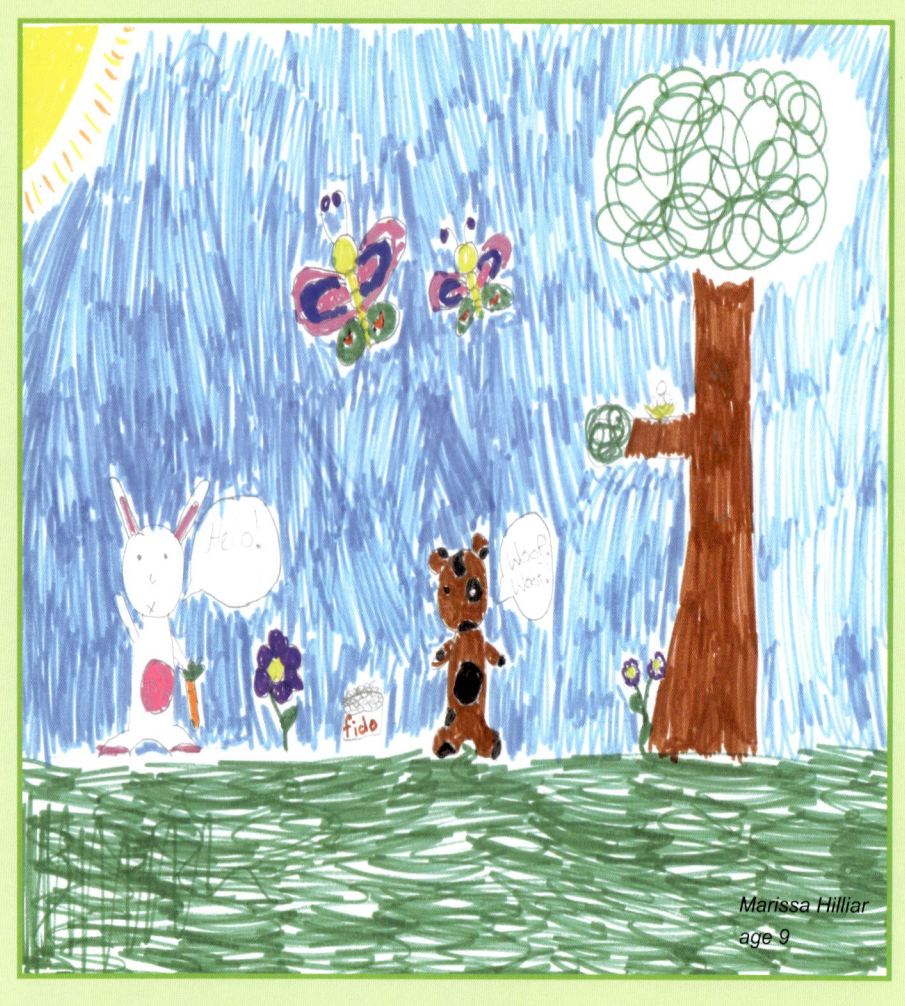

Marissa Hilliar
age 9

⭐**Riddle**

Why do golf players wear two pairs of trousers?

⭐**Answer**

In case they get a hole in one!

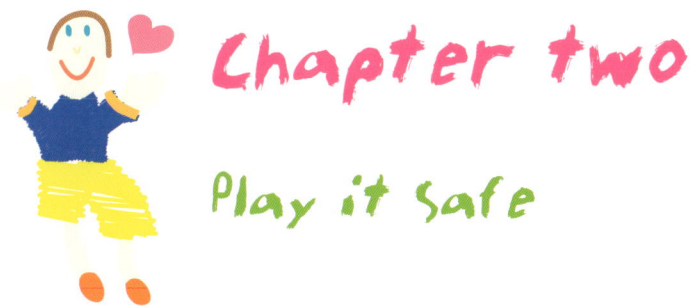

Chapter two

Play it safe

Just because essential oils are natural doesn't mean that you do not need to be careful with them. They are complex chemical mixtures of organic molecules, which must be used according to safety guidelines – if you abide by the guidelines essential oils are very safe to use.

The main safety guidelines to observe when using essential oils are:

☹ Never ingest the oils, unless you are under the direction of a qualified, registered aromatherapist.

☹ Never apply pure essential oils directly to the skin, unless specifically advised to by a qualified registered aromatherapist.

☹ Never exceed the recommended dosage; using a higher dosage does not increase the oils' effectiveness.

There have been some extreme claims made about the safety of essential oils over the years and you might read something in an older aromatherapy text that differs from what you read here. The information in this book is current at the time of printing. Most of the contraindications you will read about relate to the ingestion of essential oils, not to their external use. If you'd like to do more research yourself into the latest findings about essential oil safety, I recommend reading *Essential Oil Safety* byTisserand and Balacs and *The Complete Guide to Aromatherapy* (second edition) by Battaglia. If you are in any doubt, please consult with a qualified, registered aromatherapist.

Essential oils and pregnancy

The latest research by Tisserand and Balacs suggests that essential oils are safe to use during pregnancy, as long as they are not taken orally and that the directions for use are followed. A maximum dilution of 2 per cent is recommended for massage oils. Tisserand and Balacs say that '…the external use of camphor-rich oils such as Rosemary is safe in pregnancy'. They do suggest however that Aniseed and Fennel should be avoided during pregnancy because of their oestrogenic activity, which may influence the menstrual cycle. For more information see *Essential Oil Safety* by Tisserand and Balacs.

Safety dilutions

★ **for children**, dilute essential oils into a base of cold-pressed almond or apricot kernel oil. If the child has particularly sensitive skin, use a lower dilution.

★ **6 months to 2 years**, use 1 drop of essential oil to 10ml of base oil.

★ **2 to 5 years**, use 2 drops of essential oil to 10ml of base oil.

★ **5 to 10 years**, use 3 drops of essential oil to 10ml of base oil.

★ **10 years and over**, use 5 drops of essential oil to 10ml of base oil.

★ **for Adults,** use about 90 drops of essential oil to 100ml of carrier oil.

★ **Adults with sensitive skin**, use a total of 30 drops of essential oil to 100ml of carrier oil. (If you are using a blend of three or more different essential oils, use a total of 30 drops, not 30 drops of each oil.)

★ **Pregnant women**, use about 40 drops of essential oil to 100ml of carrier oil.

★Photosensitisation

Bergamot, Lemon and Lime essential oils, when used in any way that applies them to the skin, can increase photosensitivity, which means that your skin will become sunburnt faster. Use these essential oils with care before exposure to sunlight. Photosensitivity is not increased simply by inhaling these oils.

To get the best effects from essential oils:

☺ Don't use the same oil all of the time; you can build up a resistance to the oil and find that it becomes less effective.

☺ Synergistic blends of oils (that is, blends made up from three or more essential oils) are more effective than single oils.

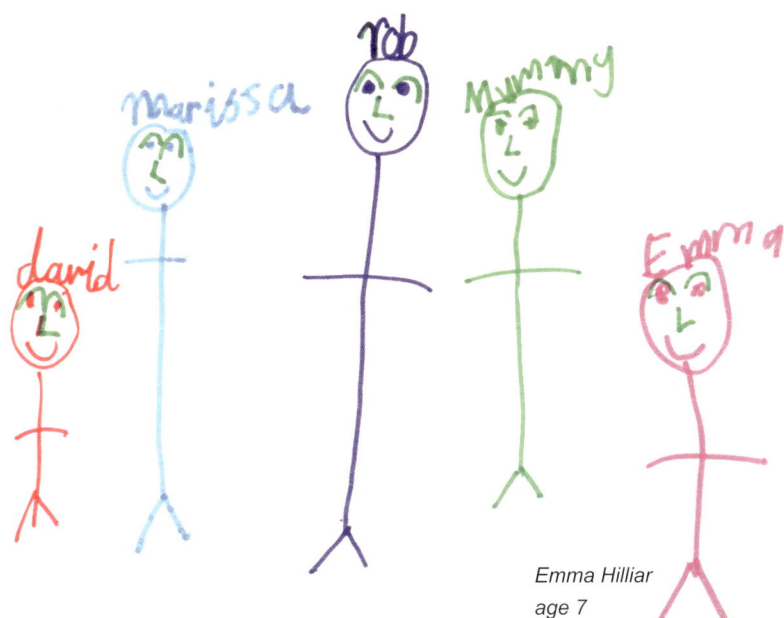

Emma Hilliar
age 7

15

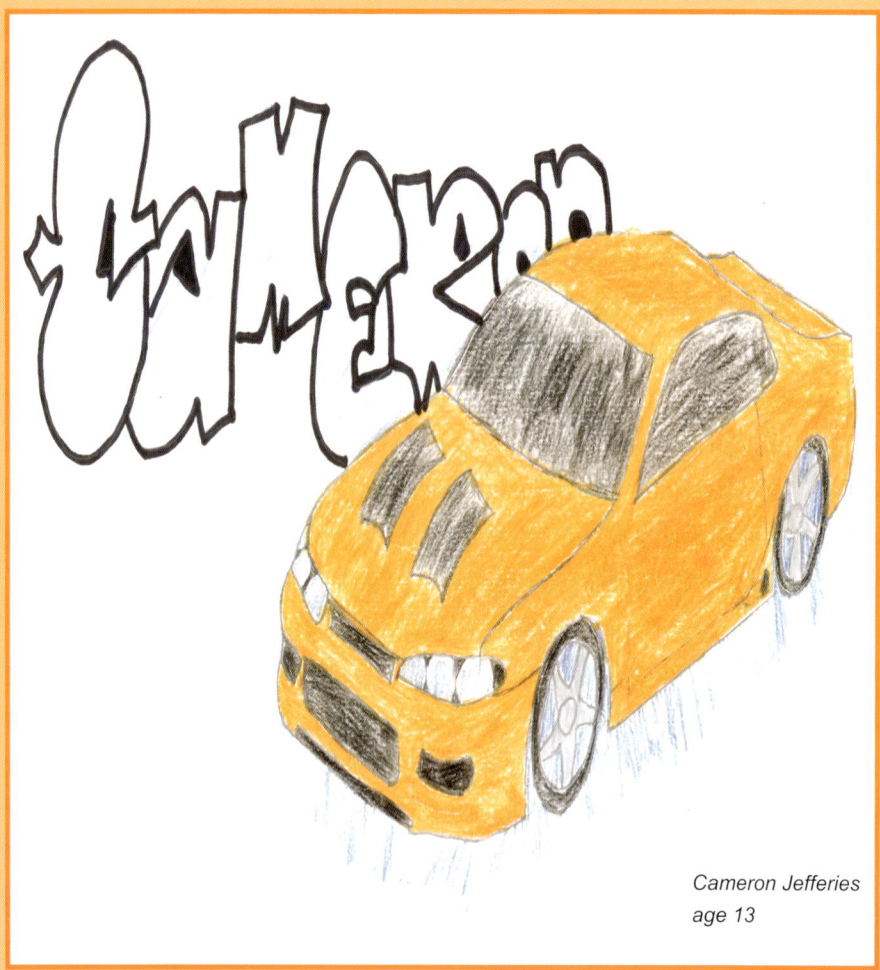

Cameron Jefferies
age 13

★ **Riddle**

Why was six afraid of seven?

★ **Answer**

Because seven eight nine!

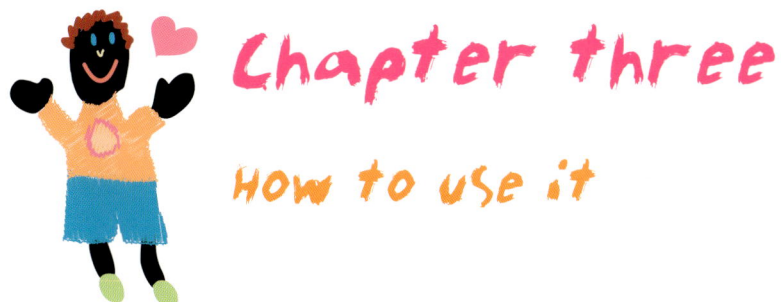

Chapter three

How to use it

There are many ways that you can use aromatherapy both as a treatment for specific ailments and injuries, as well as an integral part of your daily life to help deal with emotional upsets and issues, these include:

Oil vaporisers

I prefer to use electric oil vaporisers; they are safe, efficient and if you use the six-watt style you don't have to worry about hot water. You simply choose the essential oils you wish to use and put a total of 10 drops into the vaporiser, plug it in and switch it on. The ceramic bowl produces just enough heat to release the scent of the essential oil. (These vaporisers carry the 'C-Tick' which indicates that they do not cause interference with nearby communication or electrical equipment.) Some electric oil vaporisers have a hotter element and do require you to add water. These need constant attention to make sure that the water doesn't evaporate dry. Make sure that you know which type of electric vaporiser you have before using it.

If you prefer the romance of the candle in the traditional oil vaporisers, place a little water in the bowl above the candle, add 5-10 drops of essential oil to the water and light the candle. Never leave these vaporisers unattended where they can be knocked over, where the flame can come into contact with anything (or anyone) and never allow the water to burn dry.

All types of vaporisers can be easily cleaned by wiping the bowl with a damp sponge or towel.

When it comes to having kids in the house, I much prefer to see the electric vaporisers being used to prevent the danger of mishaps.

Inhalations

With small children an inhalation can be as simple as putting a drop of Lavender essential oil onto the front of their pyjamas or sheets at night time to help them sleep. I am not keen on putting a drop of essential oil onto a child's pillow, because they can roll onto it and the oils could cause irritation to sensitive skin. Try putting a drop onto the top sheet instead, where it is near their nose, but there's less chance of them lying on it.

You can also use the handkerchief or tissue method, which is more portable. Simply put 3-4 drops of essential oil onto a handkerchief or tissue and hold it near their nose for a few minutes while they inhale. For young children, use 1-2 drops.

If the child is old enough, add 5-10 drops of essential oil to a bowl of steaming water, place a towel over his or her head and the bowl, and have them inhale the vapours for a few minutes.

Compresses

A compress is a quick, effective, easy and practical application for essential oils. First, decide whether a cool or warm compress is appropriate.

★ Cool Compresses

For a 'hot-and-bothered' headache use a cool Lavender and Spearmint compress: add 5 drops of essential oil to 200ml of cold water, soak a cloth in the water, wring it out and place over the forehead for fifteen minutes.

★ Hot Compresses

For a 'foggy' head, sinus congestion or painful periods repeat the same method using warm water instead of cold.

Humidifiers

Essential oils can be used in humidifiers, the type we generally see has a small well in the front that the steam blows across. You can add 3 drops of essential oil to the water in the well and this will be diffused throughout the room. Some essential oils can leave a sticky residue, if you have a more complex, electric humidifier ascertain whether any essential oil residue will be a problem before you use oils in it.

Massage

Massage is considered one of the oldest and simplest of all medical treatments. It is easy to integrate regular massage into your life and it can help you to achieve and maintain good health. With massage you gain the benefits from the essential oils as they are absorbed into the skin and as you inhale the aromas. Small children love and crave touch. They spend the first nine months of their lives being cradled and caressed inside their mother's womb and once outside, it is reassuring to them to feel regular touch. A close friend, who is an acupuncturist, was explaining to me that the process of being squeezed through the birth canal switches on the baby's triple warmer and resulting immune system. Cesarean born babies do not experience the squeezing effect and require touch and massage even more importantly than others. Some new parents are afraid to massage their baby for fear of hurting them. Babies are actually quite tough and can take a firm but gentle pressure. It is important to use good quality oils to ensure no sensitisation to the baby.

To blend a massage oil, first consult the safety dilutions on page 14 to get the correct dilution for your child. Then review chapter 5 on carrier and infused oils to choose the most suitable base oil for your needs.

★Soothing Baby Massage Oil★

This recipe is a basic baby massage oil which will be soothing and calming. The oil can help to settle everything from skin irritations to nappy rash, cradle cap, teething pains and stomach aches.

- ★ 4 drops Lavender

- ★ 3 drops Tangerine

- ★ 3 drops German Chamomile

- ★ 40ml Apricot Kernel oil

- ★ 10ml Calendula oil

☺ **Please note:** Never use mineral-based oils such as baby oil as carrier oils in aromatherapy; they do not carry essential oils effectively and cause sensitivity problems for many babies and adults.

★*Aroma Tip:* Applying vegetable oils to damp skin is ideal as it seals moisture into the skin.

 20

Bath oils

Bath time for babies should be fun, and it can also be therapeutic. Even tiny babies love bath time; because they have spent so much time in their mother's tummy, which is also a fluid environment, they feel right at home.

A baby bath blend which soothes, relaxes and moisturises the skin could contain German Chamomile, Lavender and Tangerine in a dispersing bath oil base. Always use the same dilutions as for creating a massage oil. The ideal way to use essential oils in the bath is to use a bubble bath or bath oil base made from a naturally derived cleanser to dilute the oils and disperse them throughout the water. Bath oils leave a fine coating on the body that is both moisturising and therapeutic. And, when you let the water out of the bath the residue oil goes with it leaving no mess behind – and that has to make everyone happy!

Some aromatherapy books recommend adding a few drops of essential oil directly to the bath water. I am not comfortable with this as some people may have a sensitivity to the oils. Other books recommend adding essential oils to a carrier oil and adding this to the bath water. While this does dilute the essential oils, it also causes them to float on the surface of the water, so only a small amount of oil will be absorbed where it comes into contact with the skin (that is, at the top of the water). Carrier oils are also very slippery in water, and when you let the water out of the bath you will be left with a very oily mess that no one wants to clean up!

★**Herbal Tip:** For a relaxing bath, make a jug of organic chamomile tea and when it has cooled add it to the baby's bath. It is gentle and kind to the skin, as well as relaxing and calming to the baby.

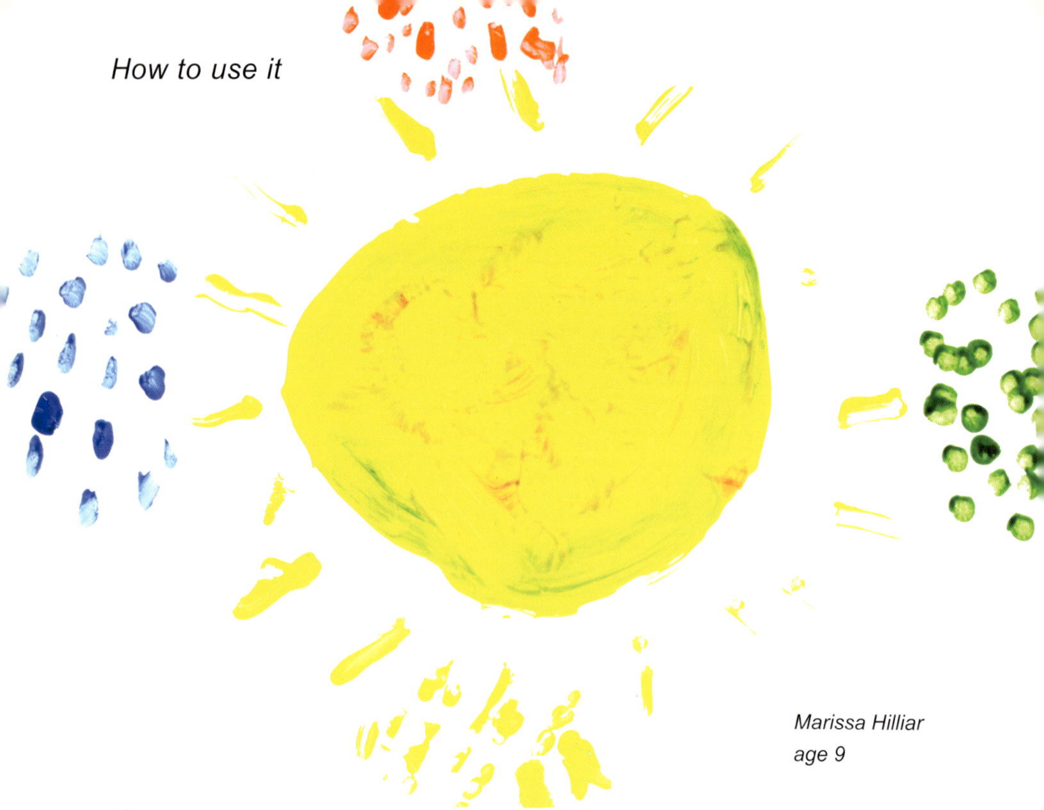

Marissa Hilliar
age 9

Soaps

A basic baby soap will generally be made using a cold-pressed vegetable oil such as jojoba, evening primrose or apricot kernel and will be infused with calendula oil for its skin healing properties. Lavender and German Chamomile essential oils make it gentle and calming on a baby's delicate skin.

Shampoo

Kids, and babies in particular, have fine hair so a gentle shampoo which is free from detergents and synthetic chemicals, colours and preservatives is essential. Coconut derived cleansing agents are available as shampoo bases for children. Essential oils such as Chamomile and Lavender can then be added to settle the child's scalp and cleanse the hair.

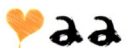

Bandages and dressings

Sometimes it only takes a bandage to make everything better. Put a single drop of Lavender essential oil onto the bandage or dressing, let it soak in for a few seconds and then cover the wound. It will assist in the healing process and soothe the emotions.

Body Sprays or face Spritzers

For those times when you can't or don't want to use a vaporiser around the home or in the car, you can prepare a quick body mist. Simply blend 50 drops of essential oil (that is, 50 drops in total, not 50 drops of each oil in your blend), 50 drops of essential oil soluboliser (which allows the oils to blend with the water rather than float on top of it) and 100ml of filtered water. Shake well, spray and enjoy.

Relaxing Shopping Spray

This is a simple way to take aromatherapy out and about with you when shopping or running errands. If your child gets wound-up or distressed, simply mist this gently on his or her face and arms to help them settle down.

★ 4 drops Lavender

★ 3 drops Lime

★ 2 drops German Chamomile

★ 1 drop Cedarwood

★ 30 drops essential oil soluboliser

★ 100ml purified water

Room freshener

You'll need a spray bottle, 100ml of filtered water, some essential oil soluboliser, and the essential oils of your choice. Blend and spray. It smells great and you receive the oils' therapeutic benefits too.

★ Happy Room Freshener ★

My favourite recipe for a harmonious, enthusiastic environment is as follows, it makes up 100ml of room spray.

★ 20 drops Bergamot

★ 20 drops Grapefruit

★ 10 drops Nutmeg

★ 10 drops Pine

★ 60 drops essential oil soluboliser

★ 90ml purified water

In the car

Road trips can be very interesting with squirmy kids in the car. Some kids find road trips of any distance upsetting and many experience travel sickness. You can use essential oils to help everyone feel more relaxed and uplifted (including Mum and Dad), and to prevent travel sickness. Essential oils such as Peppermint or Spearmint are refreshing and very effective in preventing and treating travel sickness. The only essential oil that I don't recommend being vaporised in the car is Lavender; its strong relaxing properties may prevent you from concentrating on driving. You can purchase a special car diffuser which plugs into the cigarette lighter in the car. The scent lasts for up to several days, depending on which oils you use.

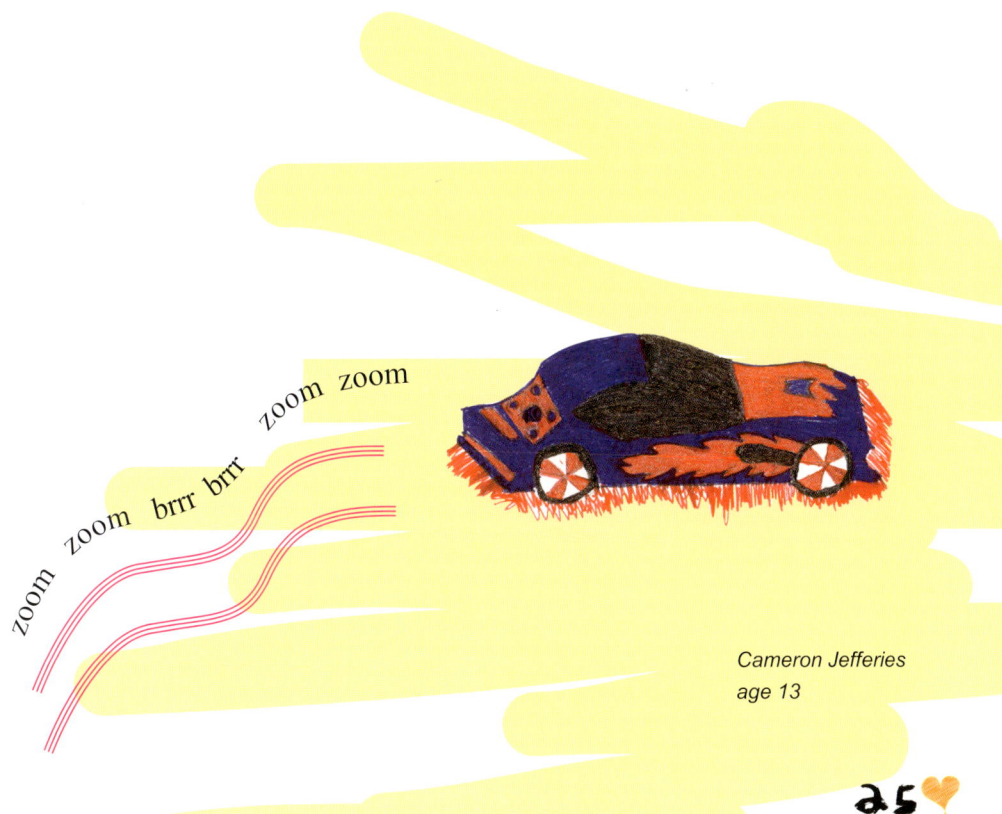

*Cameron Jefferies
age 13*

25

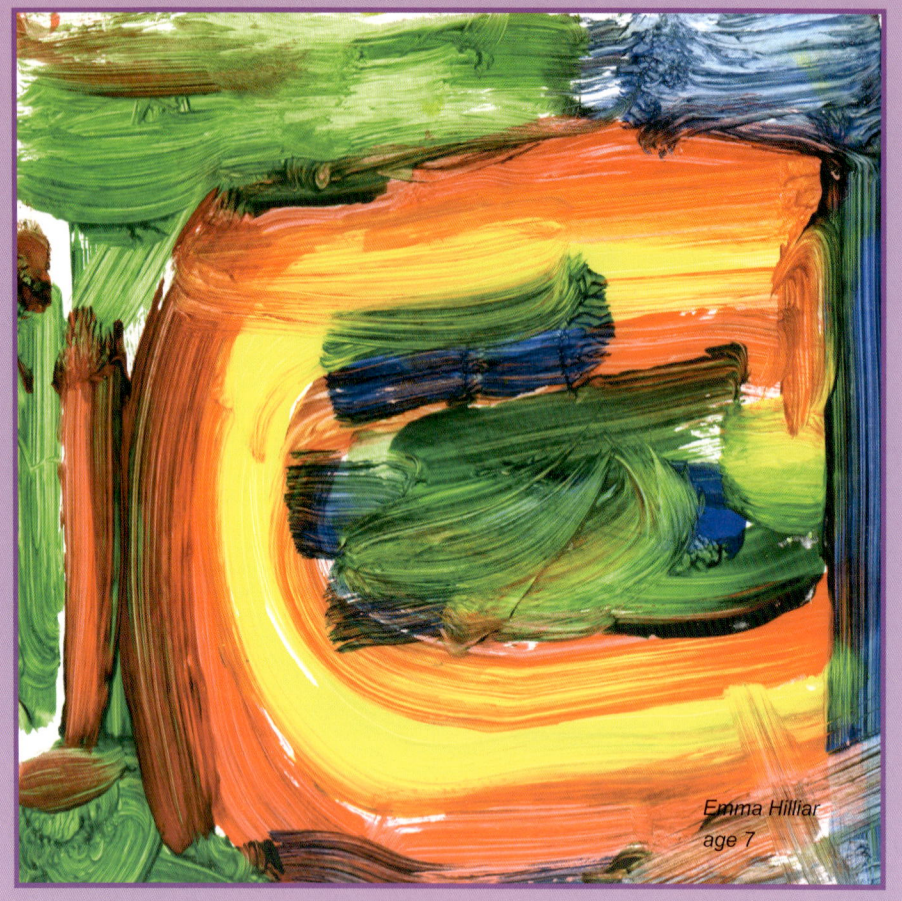

Emma Hilliar
age 7

follow your nose

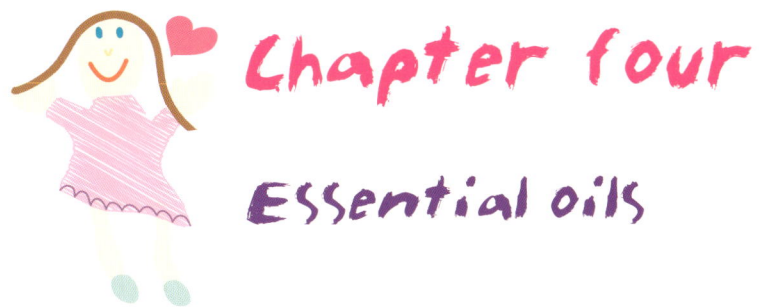

Chapter four

Essential oils

As an aromatherapist I have hundreds of essential oils at my disposal to use in my work. In this chapter I'll describe a selection of the most commonly used essential oils; these oils will provide benefits for most of the common physical ailments and emotional challenges that life presents.

Buying your essential oils

☺ The common name of the essential oil and the botanical name of the originating plant are important. The botanical name is the Latin, difficult-to-pronounce name. I have listed the Latin names of the essential oils next to their common names in this chapter. Buying essential oils based only on their common name can lead to confusion. For example, Marjoram, *Marjorama hortensis*, is a relaxant and is commonly known as Sweet Marjoram. Spanish Marjoram, which sounds more exotic, has the botanical name of *Thymus mastichana* and in fact is not true Marjoram but a species of Thyme. This oil is higher in constituents commonly found in Eucalyptus and it does not have the same relaxing properties as Sweet Marjoram; always check your botanical names.

☺ Essential oils are always sold in amber, green or blue glass bottles to protect them; do not buy essential oils in clear glass.

☺ Check the safety information listed on the packaging. Some essential oils are scheduled as poisons and should carry the appropriate warnings and advice on their labels.

☺ Look for a 'use by' date and an indication of the oil's expected shelf life.

☺ Check which part of the plant was used to manufacture the oil; different parts of the plant yield different qualities of essential oil.

☺ Always look for small print that indicates whether the oil has been diluted with Jojoba or another oil. It is reasonable for the more expensive essential oils to be diluted in Jojoba oil, but if it is diluted the label must say so. There is a big difference in price between a diluted oil and a 100% pure essential oil – look to the price to help you determine whether the oil is pure or diluted.

☺ Buy your oils from a reputable dealer, not from the local markets.

Storing essential oils

☺ Always store essential oils in a cool, dry, dark place away from heat and light. Essential oils do not like extremes – never store them in the refrigerator or in heat in excess of 30 degrees.

☺ Essential oils are volatile and will evaporate if not kept in bottles with tight lids. They are also flammable and must be kept away from naked flames. Storing your oils in a wooden box is ideal for maintaining their quality and shelf life.

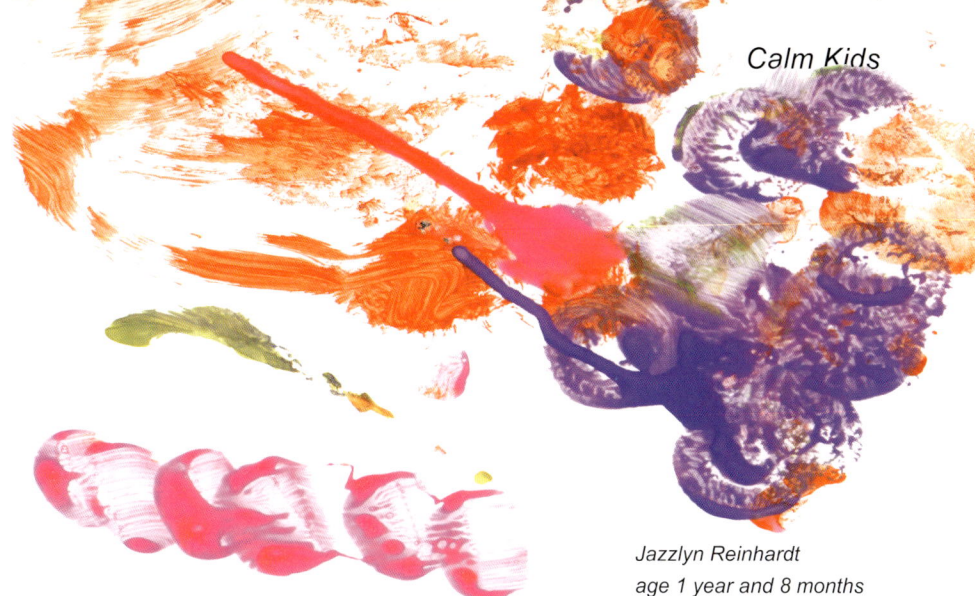

Jazzlyn Reinhardt
age 1 year and 8 months

The Essential oils

★ Basil *Ocimum basilicum*

Basil is a memory and mental stimulant. It is kind to the brain, relieving nervous exhaustion and 'life overload'; it clears the head of intellectual fatigue and brings clarity and strength to the mind. It is excellent for studying. Basil is also useful for digestive disorders such as nausea, vomiting, gastric spasms and hiccups.

★ Bergamot *Citrus bergamia*

Bergamot is a mood enhancer that uplifts and relieves nervousness. It alleviates acne and cold sores and stimulates the urinary system. It is a carminative to the digestive system and is recommended for relieving flatulence, indigestion and colic. It has a potent antiseptic action and is beneficial for treating wounds, herpes and acne. It also promotes cheerfulness.

★ Black Pepper *Piper nigrum*

Black Pepper stimulates and improves the digestive system, reducing flatulence, constipation and loss of appetite. Applying a massage oil blend that includes Black Pepper to arthritic and rheumatic aches and pains and muscular stiffness will bring a warm and reassuring relief. Emotionally, Black Pepper helps you to find your direction in life.

★ Cedarwood – Virginian *Juniperus virginiana*

Cedarwood is grounding; it relieves nervous tension and has a sedative effect. It is an astringent and antiseptic for the skin and is beneficial in treating acne, dandruff and seborrhea of the scalp. Cedarwood also relieves catarrhal conditions, bronchitis and associated respiratory disorders, cystitis and urinary tract infections. Cedarwood instills courage.

★ Chamomile – German *Matricaria recutita*

Chamomile acts as an anti-inflammatory, relieving arthritis and muscular aches and pains. It eases acne, inflamed skin and can reduce redness in the cheeks. Chamomile is also a wonderful relaxant. It is considered one of the gentlest essential oils and is especially beneficial for use with children. I have used it extensively to make anti-inflammatory and analgesic massage oils for children who are having trouble with teething. Chamomile allows you to let go of emotional worries and move on.

★ Cinnamon *Cinnamomum zeylanicum*

Cinnamon is a powerful antiseptic and one of the most potent antibacterial agents known. It is used to treat viral and contagious diseases and fungal conditions. Cinnamon is warming, giving relief to arthritic and muscular aches and pains as well as coughs and colds, nervous tension and exhaustion. It is regarded as an excellent gastrointestinal stimulant, calming digestive system spasms and ailments. Cinnamon warms your spirit and removes emotional coldness.

★ Clary Sage *Salvia sclarea*

Clary Sage is known as a euphoric essential oil. Strengthening but relaxing, it relieves nervousness, mild anxiety and emotional stress. It is one of the most important essential oils for treating women's reproductive disorders throughout all stages and cycles of life. It is renowned for relieving menstrual cramps and its antispasmodic action also makes it beneficial for treating asthma and the emotional stress that goes with it. Clary Sage provides clarity in life.

★ Cypress *Cupressus sempervirens*

Cypress is a respiratory sedative, effective in treating coughs and bronchitis. I have used Cypress in my clinic for its antispasmodic action and found it to be very effective as a preventative for asthmatics. It also strengthens an exhausted nervous system, restoring calm to life. Cypress is a menstrual regulator suitable for most women's reproductive system ailments. Cypress helps in times of emotional and physical transition.

★ Eucalyptus *Eucalyptus radiata*

Eucalyptus is best known as a decongestant inhalation used to treat colds and catarrh. It is a potent antibacterial, antiseptic and analgesic. Eucalyptus relieves muscular aches, pains and neuralgia. One drop applied to the temple can bring relief to a headache. It can be blended with Bergamot to topically treat cold sores and herpes. Emotionally, Eucalyptus removes restriction, and releases regrets and fear, helping you to be spontaneous again.

★ Fennel – Sweet *Foeniculum vulgare dulce*

Being a carminative, Fennel relieves colic, nausea, flatulence and digestive disorders. It is tonifying, detoxifying and an effective diuretic and lymphatic decongestant. It is recommended for regulating the menstrual cycle and removes feelings of being overwhelmed, bored and afraid of failure.

★ Frankincense *Boswellia carterii*

Frankincense has an affinity with the lungs; it is an antiseptic and expectorant beneficial for bronchitis and catarrhal conditions. It is a sedative that relieves anxiety, nervous tension and stress-related conditions, which makes it excellent for asthmatics whose condition is associated with nervousness. Frankincense is calming and settling, useful for meditation or when you just need to keep your feet on the ground. It is recommended for scars and wounds. Frankincense protects your space and you from worry and overwhelm.

★ Geranium *Pelargonium graveolens*

Geranium has a regulating effect on the nervous system, assisting in the reduction of nervous tension, nervous exhaustion and neuralgia.

It is a lymphatic stimulant and diuretic making it beneficial in treating fluid retention and cellulite. It is an adrenal stimulant, regulating and balancing fluctuating hormones, which in turn assists in rebalancing the moods and emotions associated with premenstrual tension. Geranium is extremely popular in skin care for its balancing effect on the production of sebum, making it beneficial for dry, oily or combination skin. Geranium is also excellent for rebalancing the extremes of life, when you're emotionally 'up' one minute and 'down' the next.

★ Ginger *Zingiber officinale*

Warming and stimulating, Ginger soothes arthritic and muscular aches and pains and diminishes digestive system disorders, bloating and flatulence. It is an effective expectorant that relieves catarrhal conditions, sore throats, coughs, sinusitis and colds. Emotionally, it releases you from procrastinating so that you can just get on with whatever has to be done, it is great to add to a study blend.

★ Grapefruit *Citrus paradisi*

Grapefruit is a light-hearted essential oil whose fragrance is uplifting to the spirit. It is valuable for treating depression, stress and nervous exhaustion. It is a lymphatic system and gall bladder stimulant and acts as a detoxifier, reducing cellulite, obesity and fluid retention. Grapefruit has a tonic effect on the scalp and skin and is an astringent. It is an effective treatment for acne and oily skin. Emotionally, it releases self-doubt and frustration amd promotes optimism and a positive attitude.

★ Juniper *Juniperus communis*

Juniper is a diuretic and detoxifier and is considered one of the best treatments for the early stages of urinary tract infections (always use common sense, if there is pus or blood in the urine, seek medical help). Juniper is recommended for skin conditions that have an accumulation of toxins, such as weeping acne, eczema and dermatitis. Juniper is also a lymphatic decongestant that works wonders in clearing toxins and reducing uric acid levels in arthritic and rheumatic conditions, gout and cellulite. Emotionally, Juniper helps you to prepare for any change that is coming in life.

★ Lavender *Lavandula angustifolia*

The 'mother' of all essential oils, for all of life's little knocks. Lavender eases cuts, scratches, bumps and bites, boils and wounds. It is commonly linked to skin care with its ability to soothe burns, including sunburn, and heal damaged skin. Acne, eczema, dermatitis, and psoriasis – any inflammatory skin condition benefits from the use of Lavender. Lavender is the preferred choice in treating insomnia, especially when it is due to mental stress or anxiety. It is anti-inflammatory and used to treat menstrual pain, and muscular aches and pains. Use Lavender to create your own 'protected space' where you can feel uninhibited and free to be all that you want to be.

★ Lemon *Citrus limonum*

Lemon is known as an excellent circulatory system tonic, helping to break-up plaque deposits in the arteries, reducing cholesterol and blood viscosity. It is antibacterial, abating infection, and is referred to as having immune stimulating properties. It is an astringent, reducing oily skin problems and its antibacterial properties lend it to the treatment of warts, boils and acne. Lemon is also mentally stimulating and removes emotional, irrational outbursts from your life.

★ Lemongrass *Cymbopogon citratus*

Lemongrass is uplifting and stimulating, it aids logical thinking and is ideal when concentration is needed. It is recommended for the treatment of sports injuries such as sprains and strains, dislocations and bruises. Lemongrass is considered to be a digestive stimulant relieving indigestion, colitis and gastroenteritis. Its antiseptic properties make it an excellent oil to vaporise when there is illness in the house. For renewed passion and excitement in your life, Lemongrass gives you that kick-start to get you going.

★ Lime *Citrus aurantifolia*

Lime is an astringent that counteracts excessive oil production in the skin. It is recommended for treating throat infections and symptoms of the flu. It is a digestive tonic that relieves general digestive ailments. Both cold-pressed and distilled Lime oil relieve a tired mind and fatigue, especially when apathy and anxiety are also present. Lime gives you the feeling that you are hanging out in a hammock and relaxing, your emotions are having a holiday.

★ Mandarin *Citrus reticulata*

Calming and refreshing, Mandarin has a tonic effect on the digestive system, calming digestion and colic. It is recommended for acne, oily and congested skin. Mandarin is considered the children's remedy; it settles tummy upsets and restlessness in 'go-fast' children. It makes an excellent addition to a pregnancy massage oil to assist in the prevention of stretch marks. Mandarin brings out your inner child to play.

★ Marjoram *Marjorama hortensis*

Marjoram is a sedative, easing nervous tension and insomnia and has the ability to strengthen tired nerves. Muscular aches and pains can benefit from Marjoram's analgesic properties. It makes an excellent chest rub for colds and flu and its antispasmodic action assists in the relief of chronic coughs. Menstrual cramps, uterine and nerve spasms are effectively calmed when Marjoram and Clary Sage are combined in a massage oil. Marjoram stops obsessive thinking and removes that negative groove from your brain.

★ May Chang *Litsea cubeba*

May Chang is a cardiac (heart) tonic that relieves the symptoms of hypertension and promotes relaxation. The essential oil has an amazingly fresh aroma that reminds me of lemon sherbet lollies. May Chang is invigorating and can alleviate the type of stress that would usually lead to depression. It is an astringent, useful for oily skin, and as a deodorant is said to reduce excessive perspiration. Use May Change to rid yourself of the 'poor me' and 'why me' mentality.

★ Neroli *Citrus aurantium var.amara*

Neroli is an antidepressant and very effective sedative that lifts the mood and guards against insomnia. It regulates heart rhythm and reduces spasms such as those experienced in nervous and stress-related heart conditions. It treats the type of nervous stomach that can lead to chronic diarrhoea. Neroli is non-allergenic and beneficial for all skin types, especially dry and sensitive skin. It helps you to make choices in life.

★ Orange *Citrus sinesis*

Children relate so well to the sweet aroma of Orange essential oil. It blends synergistically with Lavender to help children sleep and it is excellent for settling upset stomachs in both children and adults. It eases digestive system spasms and cramps, helps to expel gas from the intestines and may be used to improve the flow of bile and the metabolism of fats. Orange essential oil increases light-heartedness and relaxation, and relives nervousness and anxiety. Use Orange oil to remove the seriousness that is bogging you down in life.

★ Palmarosa *Cymbopogon martinii*

Palmarosa is used extensively in skin care and is suitable for all skin types. It has hydrating properties that help to balance oil production, promoting healthy skin and easing acne. The essential oil refreshes the moods and emotions, and may be used to settle restlessness and anxiety. Lost appetites and sluggish digestion also benefit from Palmarosa. It allows you to embrace change and let go.

★ Patchouli *Pogostemon cablin*

Patchouli is a nerve stimulant that is particularly helpful for alleviating depression and anxiety. Inhaling Patchouli can reduce nervous over-eating. It is used extensively in rejuvenating dry skin. Emotionally, Patchouli unites all levels of your life.

★ Peppermint *Mentha piperita*

Peppermint is an effective analgesic that soothes menstrual cramps and brings fast relief to headaches, muscular pains, bruises and insect bites.

It is well respected for its ability to alleviate digestive system upsets, including nausea, vomiting, diarrhoea, flatulence and stomach pains. It is an effective decongestant and expectorant used in treating respiratory disorders, such as sinus, colds and flu. Peppermint helps you to connect emotionally with your purpose in life.

★ Petitgrain *Citrus aurantium var.amara*

Petitgrain is known as the 'poor man's' Neroli. It invigorates and increases awareness, and has a stabilising effect on the nervous system. Petitgrain is recommended for nervous exhaustion and as an aid for digestion. It is known as being a beneficial tonic for the skin, helping to reduce overactive sebaceous glands, and for its deodorising properties. Petitgrain helps you to access stored thoughts and memories, staying fluid when moving between conscious and subconscious states. Use it to access the information you require to achieve success in your life.

★ Pine *Pinus sylvestris*

An excellent expectorant, Pine eases colds, flu, coughs, catarrh and sinus congestion. It is regarded as one of the most effective remedies for clearing phlegm from the lungs. Pine is an analgesic, used extensively in liniments to relieve arthritic, rheumatic and muscular aches and pains. It is also said to be as effective as Rosemary and Thyme for combating fatigue and nervous exhaustion. Pine essential oil raises self-esteem and self-worth. Time to stop rescuing others and rescue yourself; use Thyme to help you to be strong but flexible, living your own life and letting others live their own journey.

★ Rose *Rosa damascena*

Rose is considered to be effective for all areas of life: body, mind and spirit. It is a gentle but powerful antidepressant that opens the heart, releasing fear, anxiety and anger, and bringing relaxation to the soul. It regulates menstruation. In skin care, Rose is an excellent emollient, softening and hydrating the skin while cooling and soothing the body systems. Rose renews the sense of wellbeing in all areas of your life, bringing comfort and warmth to those who have grown emotionally cold. It is great for enhancing the bond between a mother and her baby.

★ Rosemary *Rosmarinus officinalis*

Rosemary is an analgesic that gives relief to arthritic, rheumatic and muscular aches and pains; it makes an excellent massage oil for stiff and tired muscles. One drop of Rosemary massaged into the temple area will bring relief to headaches. It stimulates the central nervous system and memory while reducing mental fatigue, nervous tension and exhaustion. Used in hair care, Rosemary stimulates hair growth and prevents dandruff. Rosemary stimulates you creatively and gladdens the spirit, invoking confidence to command creative energy into action.

★ Rosewood *Aniba rosaeodora*

Rosewood is brilliant for people feeling depressed, stressed and weighed down by the burdens of life. It relieves stress and anxiety and is said to have an overall balancing effect. Rosewood is used extensively in skin care and is suitable for sensitive and damaged skin, and in the treatment of acne and dermatitis. It is also used as a deodorant. Rosewood helps you to trust your sometimes unused wise feelings, heightening perceptions and enabling you to 'see past the trees' and utilise all of your senses to help you grow.

★ Sandalwood *Santalum album*

Sandalwood is an antidepressant and sedative that has a relaxing effect on the nervous system and relieves agitated emotional states. Sandalwood is well known as an effective treatment for urinary tract infections. It is used extensively in skin care for conditions where there is inflammation and a loss of moisture. Sandalwood breaks the stress cycle and allows you to go inside yourself to contemplate life. When working from inside, we have peace and the strength to see exactly how life's events really are. Sandalwood helps keep your space as your own: strong and free from other people's negative energies, so that you can operate efficiently and enjoy life.

★ Spearmint *Mentha spicata*

Spearmint is similar to Peppermint but it has a lower menthol content, which makes it less harsh on the skin and an ideal oil to use with children. Spearmint reduces mental strain and fatigue as it cools and uplifts the spirit. It is also well known as a digestive aid, alleviating disorders such as nausea, flatulence, constipation and hiccups. Spearmint invigorates all levels of our being.

★ Tea Tree *Melaleuca alternifolia*

Tea Tree's antibacterial and antifungal properties are well documented.

It is recommended for the treatment of acne, cold sores, cuts and scratches, insect bites, oily skin rashes and tinea. Tea Tree also aids respiratory disorders such as asthma, bronchitis, catarrh, coughs and sinusitis. It replaces your 'victim' mentality and feelings of 'doom and gloom' with a feeling of understanding.

★ Thyme *Thymus vulgaris*

Thyme is an antibacterial, antiviral expectorant and tonic used to treat respiratory disorders such as catarrhal coughs, lung congestion and infection, sore throats, bronchitis and asthma. It is a known nervous system tonic that aids in the relief of mental exhaustion, nervous depression and fatigue. Thyme oil eases gout, arthritic and rheumatic pain and helps sporting injuries to heal. It is also a digestive system stimulant, easing bloating and flatulence. It is a fortifying essential oil that dispels despondency and negativity, giving those who withdraw the strength to emerge with self-confidence and to overcome obstacles. It removes fears and gives the strength to feel fulfilled and worthy.

★ Vetiver *Vetiveria zizanoides*

Vetiver has the ability to ground and relax a person who is physically, emotionally and mentally burnt out. Its musky, earthy aroma draws out stress and anxiety, relieving insomnia and depression. This is the essential oil for 'go-fast' children and adults who have trouble switching their brains off and sleeping through the whole night. It is a mild rubefacient which makes it beneficial in massage oil for muscular and arthritic aches and pains. Vetiver recharges your emotional and physical energies, and supports you through life's pains. Vetiver recharges your emotional and physical energies, and supports you through life.

★ Ylang Ylang *Cananga odorata*

Ylang Ylang is an antidepressant that effectively levels the mood swings that can come with the onset of a woman's period. Ylang Ylang is a sedative that soothes the nerves and softens anger. Conditions such as high blood pressure and palpitations benefit significantly from its hypotensive properties. It is beneficial in skin care, softening and balancing the moisture in the skin. It is the 'warm fuzzy' essential oil that reunites us with our emotional, caring, nurturing, intuitive side. This is the oil for people of all sizes who have too much angry male energy.

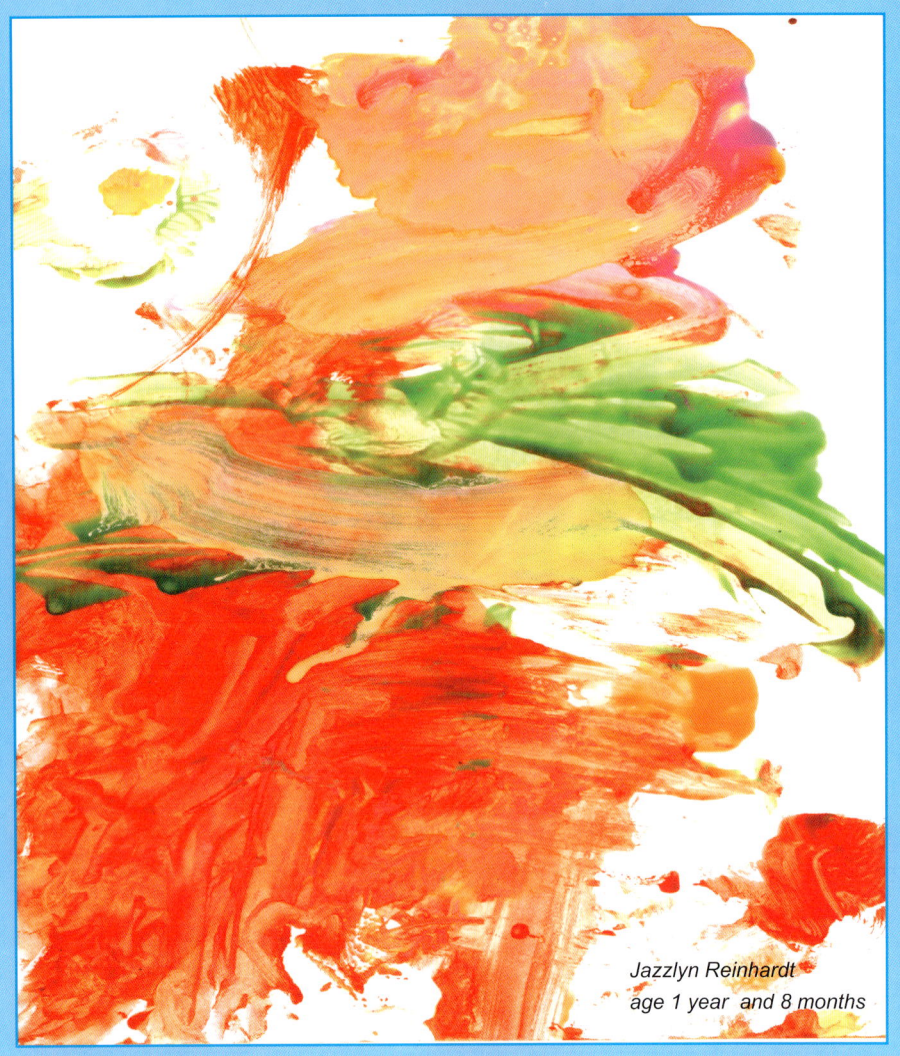

Jazzlyn Reinhardt
age 1 year and 8 months

★Young Boy: "Can I buy some bird seed, please

Pet Shop Owner: "How many birds do you have?"

Young Boy: "None, I want to grow some!" ★

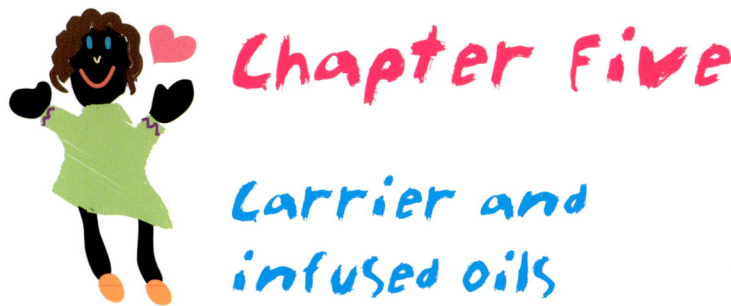

Chapter Five

Carrier and infused oils

Carrier oils, or base oils as they are also referred to, have a very important purpose. It is their job to dilute the essential oils to a safe and effective level and to enable them to be absorbed into our body systems through their fats.

When blending massage oils for children, I generally recommend a carrier oil such as almond, macadamia, apricot kernel or hazelnut. These are all finer vegetable oils which are more suitable for children's skin.

Cold-pressed oil versus cooking oil

Carrier oils should always be cold-pressed – 'cold-pressed' refers to the method of extracting the oil. When making almond oil for example, the almonds are mechanically pressed until the oil is released and it is then filtered and bottled. This oil is rich in essential fatty acids and nutritional elements. Most of the cooking oils in the supermarket are solvent-extracted. In this process the plant material is heated excessively to release the oil – it produces a much greater quantity of oil but of a far lesser quality. These oils are devoid of nutritional value and in many cases are already rancid. They are not suitable for use in aromatherapy.

Mineral oils

Mineral oils, which for decades have been marketed to mothers for use on their babies, are never used in aromatherapy. These oils have no skin penetrative properties and will not carry the essential oils through the fatty layers of the skin. The cold-pressed olive oil in your kitchen is more useful in aromatherapy than mineral oils.

The carrier oils

★ Sweet almond

Sweet almond oil has a nourishing and softening effect on the skin; it is highly nutritious, rich in trace minerals and linoleic acid, which is a polyunsaturated fatty acid. It is effective for treating skin conditions such as nappy rash, cradle cap, chafing and chapped hands.

★ Apricot kernel

Apricot kernel oil is a light oil, rich in polyunsaturated fatty acids and gentle enough to use on babies' skin. It is nourishing and makes an ideal carrier oil for cradle cap, skin chafing, nappy rash and inflamed, sensitive skin.

★ Avocado

Avocado is generally used in combination with other carrier oils. It is a rich, thick, dark green oil derived from the flesh of the avocado. Avocado oil is especially rich in vitamins A and D, lecithin and potassium. It is a heavy oil which has excellent skin penetration properties making it ideal for dry and flaky skins.

★ Evening primrose

Like avocado oil, evening primrose is generally used in blends together with other carrier oils. It is rich in fatty acids, particularly gamma linolenic acid, which makes it especially useful in assisting in the treatment of skin conditions such as eczema and psoriasis. It is also used for treating premenstrual syndrome and arthritis.

★ Jojoba

Although referred to as an oil, jojoba is actually a liquid wax, which makes it more stable than other carrier oils and very suitable for use on sensitive skin and babies. Jojoba can be used in combination with other carrier oils or on its own. It is excellent for scalp, hair and skin conditions such as eczema and psoriasis.

★ Rosehip

Rosehip oil is rich in omega-3, 6 and other essential fatty acids, making it the most superb oil for healing skin. Rosehip is used for treating conditions such as eczema and psoriasis and reducing scarring. It is generally used in combination with other carrier oils, but can also be used on its own.

★ Sunflower Seed

This is not the refined oil that you buy from the supermarket but the organic cold-pressed type. The cold-pressed oil contains essential fatty acids that are beneficial to helping the skin to heal.

★ Soybean

Soybean oil is light in texture and contains vitamin E and essential fatty acids. It is an inexpensive and effective carrier oil. Remember to purchase organic and not genetically modified oil.

★ Wheatgerm

This is the richest natural source of vitamin E. It is a heavy oil with an odour that many people find unpleasant. Its skin healing properties make it an ideal oil to blend with other carrier oils. The heavy texture and odour are masked when it is blended with other oils.

★ Dispersing bath oil

Vegetable oils can be broken down to become water soluble, and they can then be used as a base to dilute essential oils for use in the bath. A dispersing bath oil disperses the essential oils through the water and eliminates the risk of irritating sensitive skin.

★ Vegetable cream base

An unscented cream base can be used in place of carrier oils when you are treating an aliment which would suit a cream such as psoriasis or eczema. Vegetable cream bases have a texture similar to sorbolene cream but are made from cold-pressed vegetable oils and waxes, rather than mineral oils and waxes. Never use sorbolene cream in aromatherapy because it is a mineral product which cannot carry essential oils into the skin.

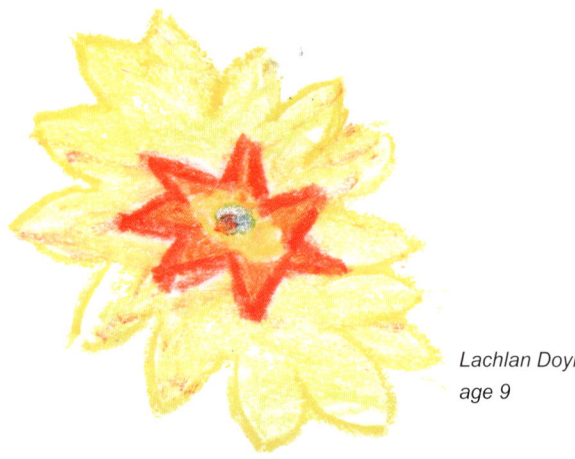

Lachlan Doyle
age 9

The infused oils

There are some plants that cannot be distilled into an essential oil nor can they be cold-pressed into a carrier oil. These are known as infused oils. They are made through the traditional process of cold infusion: herbs are immersed in cold-pressed vegetable oil and left to infuse, when complete, the oil is strained, retaining the healing properties of the herbs. Infused oils can be used either on their own or blended with other carrier and essential oils.

★ Arnica

This oil is known for its ability to release and mobilise bruising and reduce swelling. It is beneficial for sprains and strains or any soft tissue injury.

★ Calendula

Calendula oil is made from large marigold flowers and has been used for centuries as a skin healing oil. It is wonderful for everything from nappy rash to treating dry, cracked nipples from breast-feeding as well as for reducing scarring and healing the skin.

★ Carrot

Bright orange in colour and rich in vitamin A and beta-carotene, carrot infused oil brings basic skin healing properties to any blend.

★ Hypericum

Hypericum is commonly known as St John's Wort. Like arnica oil, hypericum is also used for soft tissue injuries and is beneficial for conditions such as neuralgia and shingles where pain is present in the nerve endings.

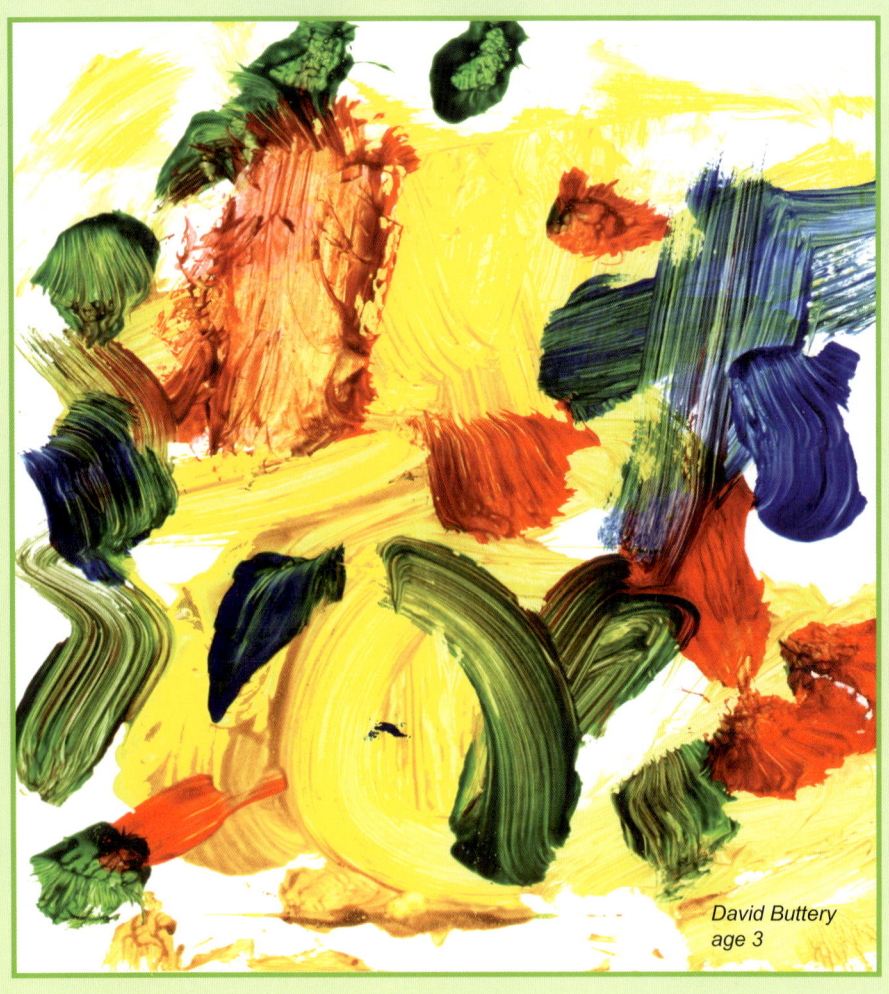

David Buttery
age 3

⭐ Riddle

What's the difference between boogers and broccoli?

⭐ Answer

Kids don't eat broccoli!

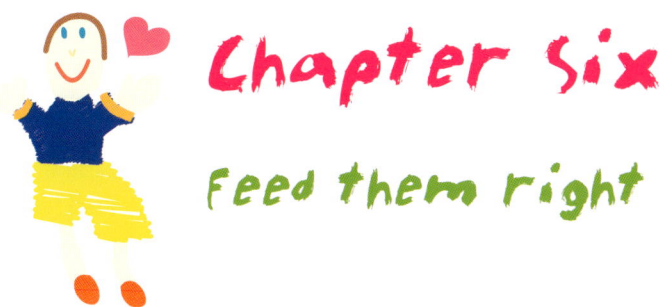

Chapter Six

Feed them right

We all know that our diet affects our wellbeing. And with children, diet is even more important because their bodies are more sensitive than adults'. There are some simple things that can be done to balance your child's diet to achieve a better state of health and a happier child.

Given the choice, most kids wouldn't choose a glass of fresh carrot juice, green vegetables, turkey breast or brown rice. Instead, they tend to focus on commercial breakfast cereals, packaged noodle soups, soft drinks and finger foods such as pizza, chips and sweets. A child's food choices are ruled by taste and texture, rather than biochemical science. The amount of dead, processed, empty food that kids eat today is unbelievable. And just like us, the more you tell them not to, the more they want it. It is only when we reach our forties that we realise if we had listened to our parents we wouldn't have to be working on undoing the imbalances that we created in our younger years! After leaving home at seventeen and joining the regular army, I remember living on litres of cola and daily take-away foods. And I loved it at the time, freedom away from Mum and Dad telling me what to eat and what not to eat – but it has taken me years to repair the damage that fun time created.

So lead by example – if you want your kids to eat healthy foods, you must eat them first and inspire them to want to do the same.

Poor nutrition negatively affects everyone emotionally, mentally and physiologically. Without optimum amounts of essential micro-nutrients, including B-complex vitamins, vitamins C and E, zinc, magnesium and chromium, young people become apathetic, moody and lose their spark for life. Food allergies and sensitivities can also be to blame. Kids are becoming more sensitive to foods because of the nutritional deficiencies in their bodies – and one of the worst offenders for draining our nutrition is the grain that we eat every day.

Bum Glue

Do you remember at school, we used to make glue out of white flour and water? Remember how it smelled after a few hours and how it set like cement when you used it? Well, that same cement-like action is happening inside your body every time you eat white breads, pasta and rice. And after it has been in there for a while, it becomes foul, sticking to the walls of your bowel and sucking the life out of you. I call it 'bum glue'.

Ideally, you should avoid grains that have had the wheatgerm removed, which is what white bread is. The germ is where most of the nutrients live. Refined and processed grains are acid-forming (high in phosphorous) and when consumed as flour, tend to cause problems in the gut (such as bloating), the brain and the joint capsules. Refined grains are also very high in phytates, which latch onto water-soluble nutrients including vitamins B and C and minerals such as calcium, chromium and magnesium. So while you could be eating what appears to be a healthy sandwich containing meat and salad on white bread, the reality is that you are not going to absorb the essential nutrients because the refined grains leach the goodness away. If you did nothing other than replace white grains with brown in your diet, your basic level of health would increase dramatically.

Most commercial wholegrain breads are made with a white wheat base and most of the supermarket rye breads, light rye in particular, are made with only about nine per cent rye flour, the remainder is primarily refined white flour.

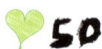

Learn to read the packaging of the foods you buy, and learn to look for hidden ingredients. Biscuits are a classic kids' food which is based on white flour 99 per cent of the time. There are some brands nowadays that are making wholemeal varieties, which are a much better alternative. Anything that you bake or buy that contains white flour can be also made using wholemeal flour, which cooks just the same, tastes great and won't glue up your body as much as white flour will – just don't tell the kids that it is good for them!

Working out which carbohydrates to eat is easy, just remember to eat unrefined brown grains (brown rice, pasta and breads) and go for low GI as well.

Psyllium husks – The unclogger

So what do you do when you realise that you have may have a little 'bum glue' stuck from years of eating refined white grains? The solution is easy. There is a grain called psyllium, it is the size of a sesame seed and you can buy the husks in the health food section of the supermarket or from the health food store. It is a wonderful raw fibre that has no taste and it makes poo bulkier, so that you can scratch off some of that gluey residue that has built up. The easiest way to take psyllium is to add two dessertspoons of the husks to a glass of juice in the morning, stir it in quickly and drink. If you let it sit in the glass it will get very thick and be very unpleasant to drink, so drink it down immediately. It has the consistency of a glass of orange juice with the pulp in it and no added taste.

In my clinic I would often see parents with kids and poo challenges. One of the suggestions I would give them was to make jelly for the kids by adding some psyllium husks to a cup of their favourite fruit juice and setting it in the fridge. When the kids eat the jelly it helps to keep them regular and to clean their digestive system at the same time. Check with your naturopath before giving psyllium to your child.

★ *Important note*: When adding psyllium husks to your diet always make sure that you are drinking your daily quota of water, the psyllium needs water to help create bulk and move the gluey bits.

Kids today are eating hundreds of kilograms of refined white flour, white rice and sucrose every year, and that's enough processed high-glycemic carbohydrate to destroy anyone's insulin metabolism. High-glycemic carbohydrates are refined and processed foods that cause the body's blood sugar to rise too fast, resulting in the body over reacting. It stimulates excess insulin causing energy levels and moods to ride a roller coaster. By middle age, or even earlier, this can lead to the development of adult onset diabetes and obesity.

Don't think that because kids are young the quality of the food they eat doesn't matter; it is vital. Over time, processed foods such as hamburgers, soft drinks and ice cream damage them on the inside. And with the sedentary lifestyle many kids now lead, instead of burning it off, it burns them out. The quality of the food kids eat today, particularly when it comes to proteins, carbohydrates and good fats, will determine the outcome of their health and body weight later in life.

People often ask me how to remember what is a protein and what is a carbohydrate – it's easy. If it comes from an animal product or legume then it's a protein, for example red and white meats, fish, dairy, soy products, etc. If it comes out of the ground, then it's a carbohydrate, for example whole grains such as bread, rice, pasta, potatoes, etc. And the rest of the whole-foods are your fruits and vegetables. So aim for a balanced portion of each at every meal and you will notice the difference.

Basic Nutrients

When it comes to kids' health there are a few basic nutrients to keep in mind. My work in clinic has shown me that antioxidants such as zinc and vitamin C, water and essential fatty acids (especially omega-3) are essential to help prevent day-to-day ailments and to maintain good health. This is because a lot of the fresh foods we eat today do not have the same nutritional content that they had in the past. Sadly our soil is devoid of many nutrients.

★ Zinc and vitamin C

The most common complaints we see in clinic these days are behavioural, with many children having difficulty settling down. Diet can influence this, specifically the intake of zinc and copper-rich foods. In ADD and ADHD children, if we do a hair tissue mineral analysis we find that they generally have a high lead content, low zinc and high copper. This imbalance generally presents with people having trouble settling. The lead imbalance is common in both children and adults. Living on a busy road, in a house with old lead paint or even chewing on a lead pencil as a habit can influence lead levels in the body. Vitamin C is an effective detoxifier for mobilising lead out of the body. Check with your naturopath to see if lead is having an affect on your child's health and for an individual dosage. Also, look at eating more zinc-rich foods such as seafood, nuts and seeds especially brazil nuts, almonds and pepitas (pumpkin seeds), and eating less copper-rich foods such as chocolate and grapes. In clinic I would always see a lot of 'go-fast' kids when the copper-rich green grapes were in season. As much as grapes are healthy for you they still need to be eaten in balance with other foods. Chocolate is also loaded with copper which can make kids go faster than the sugar content will. A high copper to zinc ratio tends to make you a little 'go-fast' and manic, while a low copper to zinc ratio tends to drop your moods and make you a little sad and teary. Again, check with your naturopath for a correct dosage for your child.

★ Water

Water, in particular filtered water, is essential to life. Our bodies are literally made up of 60-70 per cent water. Your muscles are 75 per cent water, your blood is around 83 per cent water and your bones are 22 per cent water. And because they generally have more muscle, men have a higher water content than women. Now does it make sense why everyone keeps telling you to drink more?

Water is fundamental to our body chemistry, among the most important roles it plays are keeping your body and brain hydrated. Your brain is the first place that you lose water from when you become dehydrated and this affects your ability to think straight. Water is also essential for helping your body eliminate wastes, including the acidic wastes released during times of physical or emotional stress.

☺ **So how much do you really need?** For adults, I recommend two litres of filtered water per day; this is how much an active person needs just to prevent dehydration. For kids, the following table gives you an easy calculator.

Hollday-Segar Fluid Requirement Calculation	
Weight*	**Baseline Daily Fluid Requirement**
1 to 10kg (2.2 to 22lbs)	100ml per kg
11 to 20kg (23 to 4lbs)	1000ml plus 50ml/kg for each kg over 10kg
Over 20kg (over 44lbs)	1500ml plus 20ml/kg for each kg over 20kg
*1 kg = 2.2lbs, 1 ounce =29.6ml	
Example: 30lb child	
Convert to kilograms	=30lbs / 2.2kg/lb = 13.6kg
Choose formula from above	=1000 ml + (50ml/kg x 3.6kg)
Calculate	=1000ml + 180ml = 1180ml fluid daily
Convert to ounces	=180ml / 29.6ml/ounce = 39.8 ounces fluid daily

Fluid Requirements for Children, Jennifer Murphy, http://faculty.olin.edu/~jcrisman/Service/KWTWebNews/Nutrition/fluid.htm

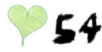

☺ **Does it have to be filtered water?** Water is potentially contaminated with toxic industrial chemicals such as chlorine, as well as nasty bacteria and heavy metals, so yes, filtered is better.

☺ **Are we talking about water specifically or just fluids?** By water, I mean water and although cordial, soft drinks, juices, tea and coffee all contain some water, the body has to process the contents of the drink before it is able to make use of the water. So water means water or herbal teas. Green tea, which has become very popular, also counts as water intake – but make sure that it is brewed for less than one minute; this way you get all of the essential antioxidants without excess tannin. Tannins are nature's waterproofing and preserving agents, they're used to turn animal hide into leather. Drink too much tea, especially the way Westerners drink it – strong and black – and you'll be drying out your insides.

If you or the kids are getting a little rattled, you may be dehydrated, so grab a drink of water.

★ Good fats

Speaking of dehydration, you can also become 'oil dry'. I mentioned earlier about good fats, such as omega-3 essential fatty acids. These are the oils that come from cold water fish and flaxseeds. Fats are the most concentrated source of energy in your diet. They also carry fat-soluble vitamins such as A, D, E and K around our bodies. It is the fats in our diet that give us that satisfied, full sensation after a meal.

There are two main types of fats. The first are saturated fatty acids, which set hard at room temperature such as the fats in meats and dairy foods. The other type are unsaturated fatty acids, which are liquid at room temperature, these are mainly found in nuts, seeds, olives, avocado and so on. There are three essential fatty acids, which are classified as unsaturated fats. These are essential for normal growth, healthy blood, arteries and nerves. They also help to transport bad fats, like cholesterol, out of the body. Cholesterol is actually important for a healthy body, but like everything in life, an excess is not good for you.

A deficiency in fatty acids can present itself as eczema or other skin disorders in people of all ages. Kids that have been labeled as ADD, ADHD or with learning disorders or behavioral problems generally also have a deficiency in omega-3 essential fatty acids and have benefited enormously from taking a supplement. The easiest way I have found to get kids to take essential fatty acids is to add a teaspoon of omega-3 from flaxseed oil into a fruit and honey smoothie. The oil blends with the milk fats and creates a yummy snack, and all the kids can taste is the fruit and honey. They will never know the difference, but you will as their behaviour changes. Consult your naturopath for a specialised dose for your child.

Suggestions for school lunch boxes:

You can pack the kids off to school with a healthy lunch but you cannot always stop them from that timeless lunchtime tradition of swapping. But, the more interesting you make their lunch, the less chance there will be of them being tempted to trade it. These are a few hints I give to parents to make lunchboxes healthier and more interesting.

★ Kids aren't always into brown sliced bread, so try a wholemeal tortilla wrap instead. It's more fun and you can load it with all of the usual healthy fillings such as chicken or turkey, salad and low fat cheese.

★ Speaking of cheese, cut cubes of real low fat cheese instead of highly-processed cheese slices.

★ Add orange wedges or fruits that are easy to eat such as mandarins and bananas.

★ Low fat yogurt is also a great lunchtime filler, give them plain yogurt and a small container of raisins, sultanas or chopped fruit to add in themselves. This avoids the added sugars that the flavoured yogurts have.

★ Cute vegetables such as cherry tomatoes and sweet red capsicum slices are always a hit and baby carrots are far more fun to eat than carrot sticks.

★ 100 per cent fruit juice with no added sugar is far superior to diluted fruit drinks.

★ I love peanut butter and so do kids, have a go at filling celery sticks with it and top them with sultanas or raisins, tell them it's called 'ants on a log'.

★ Lastly, remember the all-important water bottle. Most schools let kids have a water bottle in the classroom nowadays, which is fantastic. It is so different to when I was growing up. It is also very trendy to carry a water bottle, so that makes it easier to get them to do it as well.

After School Snack

My favourite after-school snack for kids is a fruit smoothie. Simply blend together their favourite fruit, such as a banana with some low fat milk (it can be flavored if you want) and honey. Also, add one teaspoon of flaxseed oil to make sure they are getting their daily essential fatty acids.

Kids will eat anything providing that you make it a little fun and don't tell them that it's good for them. If they are being really fussy eaters, take them to see your naturopath because sometimes this can be an indication of low nutrient levels.

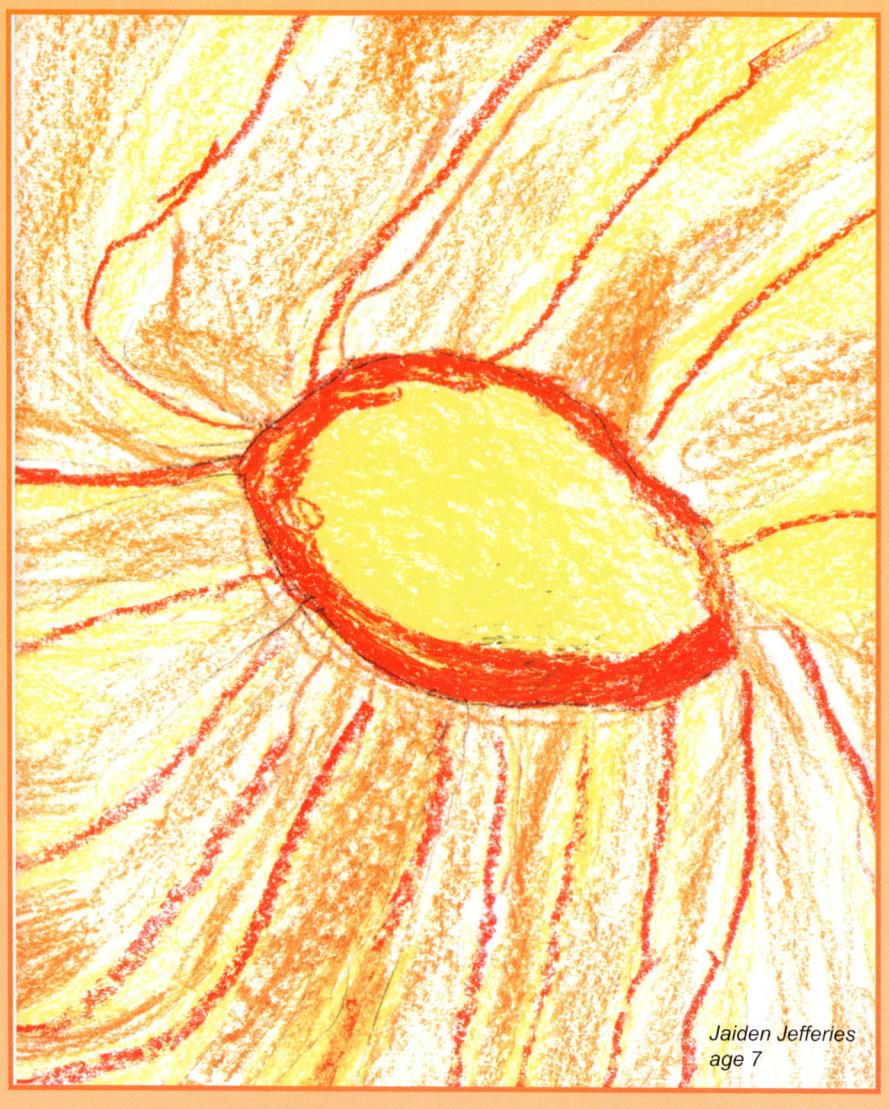

Jaiden Jefferies
age 7

We learn from experience, a man never wakes up his second baby just to see it smile.

Grace Williams

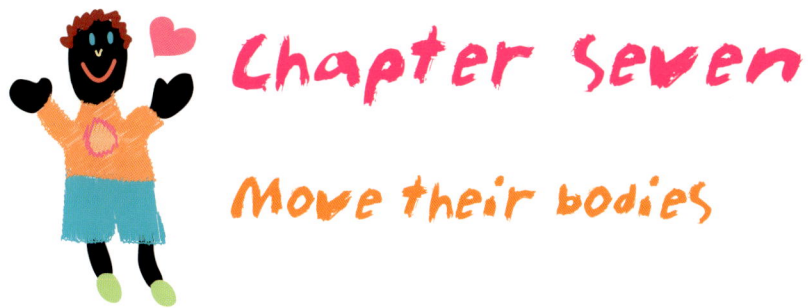

Chapter Seven

Move their bodies

I remember when I was a kid being forever outside. If we weren't racing down to the creek to catch tadpoles and guppies, we were off playing cricket or footy in the neighbour's backyard. Today things are a little different and kids aren't out and about as much as we were then. It seems to be more acceptable today for people to lead sedentary lives, and for many, the habit is forming at a very young age. As a parent, you are a primary role model in your children's lives, what are they learning from you? Many children are simply mirroring the behaviours they observe in their parents, and they're spending less and less time building forts, playing backyard cricket and catching guppies and more time in front of a computer or television.

Leading a sedentary life destroys the immune system, it robs the body of vital capacity and kills almost all of our motivation. Our bodies were designed to move, without movement, there is no life. You might feel like you move a lot – you get up every morning, get the kids ready for school, go to work, prepare meals, rush the kids around to different activities, mix with friends, go to movies, even take the family to the park on the weekends, which is all good stuff, but the quality of physical movement required to keep you healthy simply isn't there.

Move their bodies

Computers and television are not bad, they both make great babysitters, provide excellent entertainment and can even be educational. But what we need in life is balance. Too much of anything can negatively affect our health. Long hours perched in front of the monitor or big screen lends itself to physical stagnation, especially television because it also encourages overeating and the consumption of junk food.

You know how you have to take the dog for a walk? Well, the kids need to be taken for a walk and run too. Without exercise, dogs get lazy and fat, and guess what, kids are no different. Today, children are five kilograms heavier at the age of ten than they were ten years ago. Obesity is a modern plague. Excess body fat, caused by a combination of poor nutrition and inactivity, increases the risk of every disease and leads to an early grave. Keeping kids lean, fit and well nourished is essential. Their health is more often a reflection of our own efforts and personal standards, than their genetics.

Encourage children to go outside to play as often as possible. Up to the age of three or four, the best exercise is natural movement achieved through running, chasing, digging, climbing and playing at the park. When they're a little older, teach your children how to ride a bike, scooter or to roller skate. Swimming is excellent, whether at the pool or the beach.

I remember going to the beach as a kid and never wanting to get out of the surf. We would go home exhausted but incredibly happy and settled for the next week. Organised classes such as dance lessons, gymnastics and martial arts can be excellent because they teach co-ordination, emphasise stretching and can become part of your child's or family's lifestyle. If your child doesn't enjoy organised activities, that's okay too, just as long as they do some form of exercise every day. Kids have energy to burn, and if you don't get them to do something to channel that energy out, they will go a million miles an hour around the house.

For all the same reasons that your child should keep active, so should you. Be the role model you want your children to listen to and follow. If a child lives in a health conscious environment, that child will be influenced in a positive way and sadly the reverse is also true. Children's lives are a testimony to our commitment, and what more could any parent ask, than to see their children and grandchildren grow up in excellent health and live rich and fulfilling lives.

Kids can teach us a lot, besides being smaller and somewhat less confused about life, kids differ from adults in two ways: their primary purpose in life is to have fun, explore and play; and they still know how to enjoy life and laugh a lot more than we do. As adults we need to be more childlike and remember to laugh and play, instead of being boring 'grown-ups' all of the time.

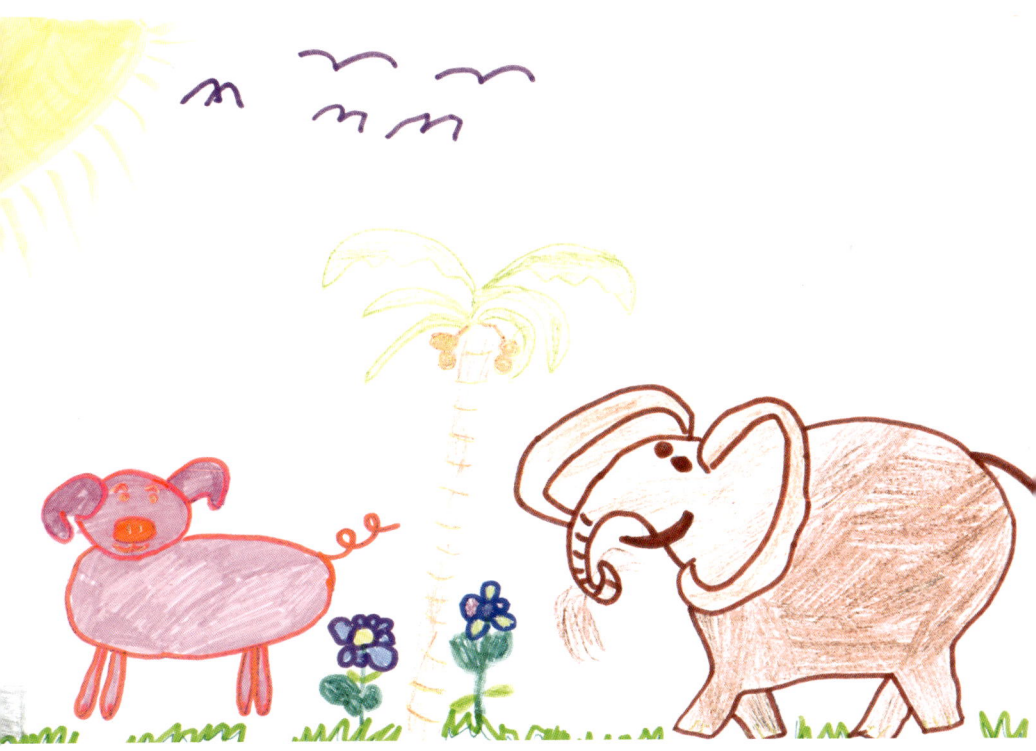

*Cameron and
Jaiden Jefferies
ages 13 and 7*

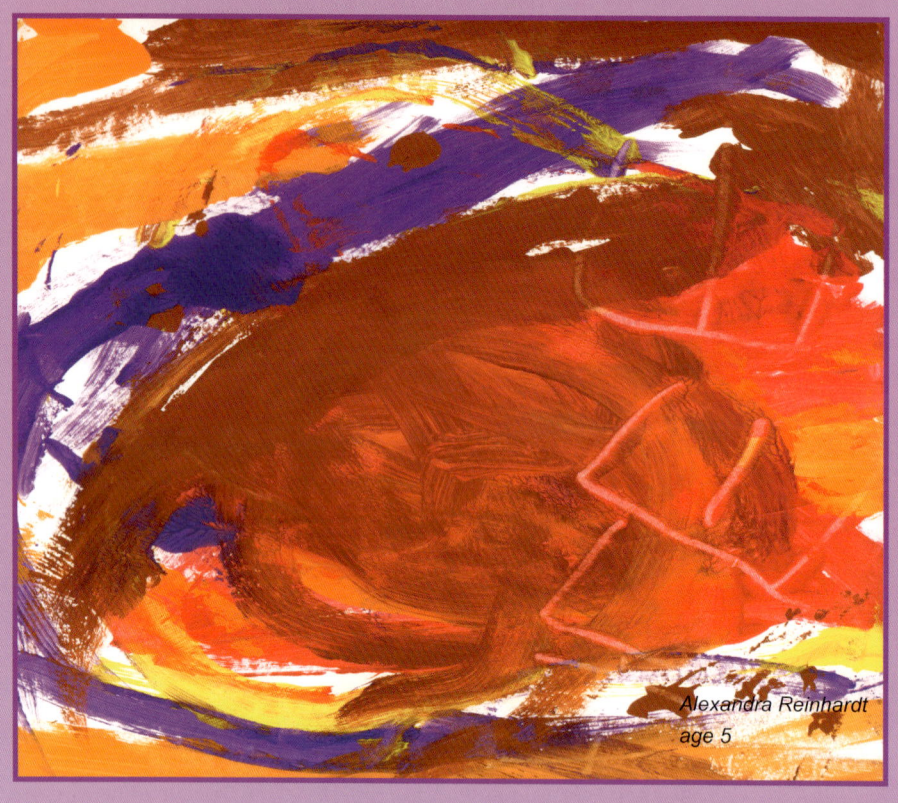

Alexandra Reinhardt
age 5

How many old nursery rhymes have been updated?

Humpty Dumpty sat on the wall,

Humpty Dumpty had a great fall.

He didn't get bruised, he didn't get bumped,

Humpty Dumpty bungee jumped.

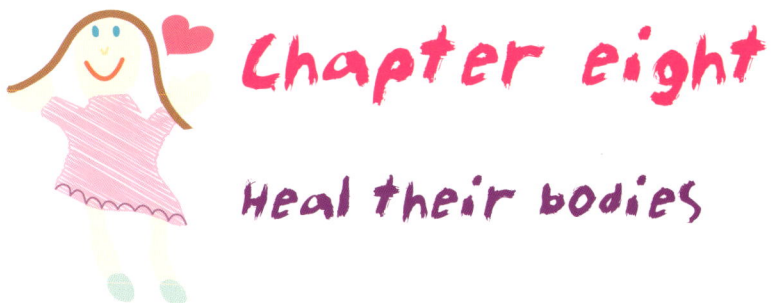

Chapter eight

Heal their bodies

In my naturopathic clinic I have seen just about every ailment a child could present with. The following is a compilation of the most common childhood ailments that I have seen and treated over the years. Because my specialty is aromatherapy, I have made suggestions for aromatherapy essential oil recipes that you can create and use, based on ways that I have treated these conditions. Use this as a guide but remember to also use common sense and seek the advice of a professional naturopath, aromatherapist or medical practitioner if needed.

These recipes can all be used in massage, bath or vaporisers.

☺ To create a vaporiser blend, simply use the recommended drops of essential oils in your vaporiser without the base oil.

☺ To make a bath oil, replace the vegetable oil with a dispersing bath oil base.

ADD / ADHD

I prefer to call these 'go-fast' kids. I worry about the medications that are being given out so frequently these days to kids all around the world.

I recently read a newspaper article that claimed that 25 per cent of boys in primary school in the United States are on Ritalin, and that the girls in the class now hold the highest academic positions. Drugs are not the answer; nutrition plays a large part in ADD (refer to page 56 for nutritional tips and consult with your naturopath for further guidance), as do emotional and environmental influences. What is certain is that these kids' behaviours do need to be addressed. They don't always understand themselves why they are behaving the way they are and it can be just as disturbing for the child as it is for the adult caring for them. One important lifestyle change is to make sure that the child has a routine to fit into – avoid big surprises or changes in their lives.

It's not only the 'go-fast' kids that you need to watch, adults can be just as fast-moving and aromatherapy is wonderful to help create a calm, positive environment for the whole family to relax in. One of the most effective things that I do as a 'go-fast' adult is use Vetiver essential oil every day. Vetiver is known for its grounding effects, it is beneficial for mental exhaustion and helps to relax a scattered mind. I use it in combination with Patchouli, Ylang Ylang, Sandalwood and Geranium, in what I call my 'Sanity Saver' blend. The way I use it in my office is in a room vaporiser and before I go to sleep I rub a few drops diluted with body oil into the soles of my feet or abdomen for a good night's rest. Vetiver is not a sedative, it simply grounds you so that you can focus on one thing at a time rather than trying to do ten things at once and not achieving anything other than driving your stress levels through the roof. It's about focusing and recharging. And at night, it helps your mind to stop racing so that you can get a good night's sleep.

The Vetiver oil in my Sanity Saver blend was used in a three-year study conducted with children suffering from ADD/ADHD. Whenever the kids felt 'scattered' they simply inhaled the oils and it was found that this settled their brainwaves back into normal patterns and improved their scholastic performance and behaviour. The results were: Lavender increased performance by 53 per cent, Cedarwood increased performance by 83 per cent and Vetiver increased performance by 100 per cent.

Over the years I have had many schoolteachers use the following essential oil blend in their classrooms to help ground kids after they've been racing around at lunchtime. I have also encouraged parents and carers to put a drop of this blend onto the soles of the child's feet to ground them so that they can sit and focus on their homework or other quiet activities.

★ Calm Kids Blend ★

When they can't settle because their minds are going so fast, ground them so they can function like everyone else. Try the following blend with a base oil for massage to rub onto your child's feet or without the base oil in a room vaporiser.

★ 2 drops Cedarwood

★ 1 drop Sandalwood

★ 3 drops Vetiver

★ 2 drops Bergamot

★ 5 drops Patchouli

★ 50ml Almond oil

Asthma

Asthma is the reversible narrowing of the bronchioles (small air tubes) as a result of inflammation of the mucous membranes or contraction of the muscular walls of the diaphragm, which results in difficulty in breathing; wheezing and coughing will occur if excessive mucous is present. Please be realistic, if your child is having an asthma attack, don't just give them some essential oils to smell – get their medication to them immediately.

Use the essential oils as a preventative; don't wait for them to get worked-up. I have had young children as clients and sent them off to school with their own blend of oils to wear on their collar enabling them to keep their respiratory system relaxed throughout the day. Try the following blend in a base oil as a chest rub or without the base oil in a vaporiser or as an inhalation.

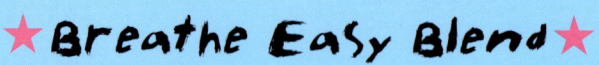

★ Breathe Easy Blend ★

Rub this blend onto your child's chest.

- ★ 4 drops Cypress

- ★ 1 drop Clary Sage

- ★ 2 drops Eucalyptus

- ★ 1 drop German Chamomile

- ★ 2 drops Frankincense

- ★ 2 drops Peppermint

- ★ 50ml Apricot Kernel oil

Athlete's foot

Especially during summer, we see lots of interesting fungal things which thrive in warm, moist conditions. Athlete's foot (also known as tinea) is infectious to the extent that is it pointless just treating a person's feet – their shoes and socks must also be treated. Tea Tree oil will break the fungal cycle, add a few drops to the washing and wipe out shoes with a few drops on a damp cloth.

★ Gumby Feet Oil ★

Massage this oil onto clean, dry feet at night.

- ★ 5 drops Tea Tree
- ★ 3 drops Patchouli
- ★ 2 drops Lemon
- ★ 20ml Calendula infused oil
- ★ 30ml Apricot Kernel oil

★ Gumby Feet Footbath ★

Bathe the feet and dry well.

- ★ 2 drops Tea Tree
- ★ 3 drops Patchouli
- ★ 100ml water

★ Gumby Feet Foot Powder ★

Sprinkle on feet during the day to absorb excess perspiration and moisture.

- ★ 8 drops Tea Tree

- ★ 8 drops Patchouli

- ★ 4 drops Lemon

- ★ 100 g green clay or talc base

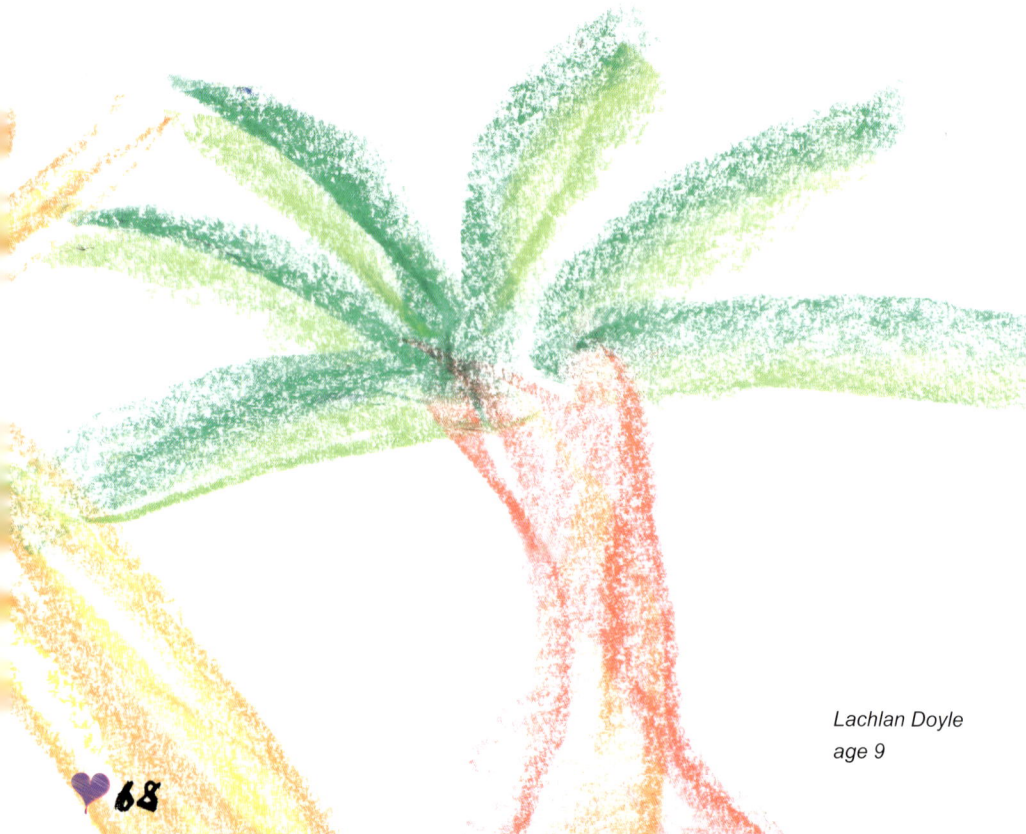

Lachlan Doyle
age 9

Bites and Stings

Common sense says to first remove the sting if possible. If the child has an allergy to the critter that has bitten or stung them, get them to a doctor to be checked immediately. Sometimes allergic reactions to bites and stings can come out over the next 24 hours, so keep an eye on the person involved (whether they are big or small). If there is no suspicion of the bite or sting being dangerous to the child's health, use the following procedure.

★ Bites and Stings First Aid ★

★ First, flush the area with cold water. If there is a chance of possible future infection, bathe the area with a few drops of Tea Tree oil in water.

★ If the area looks hot, red, inflamed or hive-like, make a cool wet compress with 5 drops of Lavender and 5 drops of German Chamomile.

★ If the area looks like it needs to be covered, place a drop of Lavender oil onto a sterile dressing and wait for it to dry before covering the wound.

Boils

These are nasty and painful eruptions that can occur anywhere on the body. Naturopathically, we have to treat them internally with herbs as well as externally; seek the advice of your naturopath for the appropriate internal treatment. For the external, aromatherapy is very useful.

Boils are pus-filled eruptions that sit below the surface of the skin; do not squeeze them. They will eventually work their way to the surface and burst. If the boil is still closed, use a few drops of a soothing oil such as Lavender or Chamomile in a warm to hot compress or bath. If the boil has burst, and the pus is coming out of the wound, you need to be careful to not infect any other area by spreading the pus.

★ Soothing Wash ★

Bathe the area twice daily with:

★ 2 drops Lavender

★ 3 drops Tea Tree

★ 2 drops German Chamomile

★ 50ml warm water

★ Calming Compress ★

- ★ 2 drops Lavender

- ★ 3 drops Tea Tree

- ★ 2 drops German Chamomile

- ★ 50ml warm water

- ★ 1 tablespoon Epsom Salts

★ Boil Dressing ★

Place the essential oil drops on a band-aid and let them dry for a few minutes before applying to the skin.

- ★ 1 drop Lavender

- ★ 1 drop Lemon

If you see a red 'poison line' running away from the boil, see a medical practitioner immediately.

Bronchitis

Bronchitis is the inflammation and/or obstruction of the bronchi (breathing tubes) that lead to the lungs. Symptoms can include coughing and expectoration, fever, back and chest ache, sore throat and difficulty breathing. Acute bronchitis usually follows an upper respiratory system infection (cold/flu) whereas chronic bronchitis results from frequent irritation of the lungs. The most effective essential oils to use in the treatment of bronchitis are: Cypress, Basil, Cajeput, Atlas Cedarwood, Aniseed, Ginger, Myrrh, Sandalwood, Thyme, Clary Sage, Eucalyptus, Pine, Lavender, Chamomile, Lemon, Frankincense, Mandarin and Peppermint.

★ Bronchitis Chest Rub ★

Use as required to help settle the symptoms of bronchitis. This blend can also be used to create a dry inhalation – do not use over steam. For kids over the age of twelve, double the drops of essential oils.

To use in a vaporiser, use the same essential oils without the base oil.

★ 3 drops Cedarwood

★ 2 drops Myrrh

★ 1 drop Thyme

★ 3 drops Frankincense

★ 2 drops Peppermint

★ 50ml Apricot Kernel oil

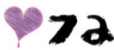

Bruises

Kids are always going to get bumps and bruises in life and Arnica infused oil loves to work on them. If a child is bruising too easily, it can be a sign of low vitamin C levels. Try a vitamin C supplement or Arnica homoeopathic tablets which are available from health food stores.

★ Bruise Healer ★

Initially use a cold compress to reduce the internal bleeding, then apply a small amount of the following blend to the bruise.

★ 6 drops Rosemary

★ 2 drops Lavender

★ 4 drops German Chamomile

★ 6 drops Black Pepper

★ 50ml Arnica infused oil

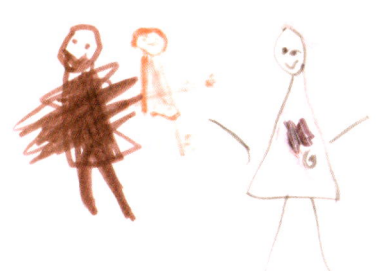

Alexandra Reinhardt
age 5

Burns

On burns, essential oils are used either undiluted or diluted into pure aloe vera gel. Use common sense, if it is a burn that needs to be seen by a medical practitioner, go immediately. Otherwise, in the first instance run the affected area under cold water for at least five minutes. Then, if the child does not have particularly sensitive skin and if the skin is not broken, apply enough Lavender oil undiluted to place a fine layer of oil over the affected and surrounding areas.

★ Burn First Aid ★

★ Burns need to be kept clean, so cover with a sterile dressing.

★ Place 3 drops of Lavender onto the dressing, allow it to dry and then cover the burn.

★ If there is a blister, never burst it, the area underneath the blister is sterile.

★ Treat the area in the same way as described above and replace the dressing daily; the blister will eventually dry and the skin will naturally heal and peel.

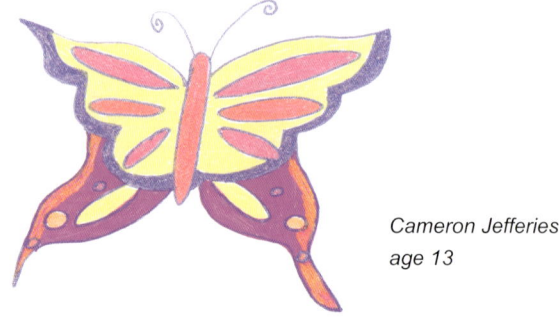

Cameron Jefferies
age 13

Catarrh (Snot)

Catarrh is the fancy name for the good old-fashioned snot that collects in the nose and/or throat. Snot happens because the body is trying to eliminate an excess of toxins (caused by diet or environment) from the mucous membranes or because of a faulty elimination of toxins by the body's eliminating systems such as the liver. Essential oils will help to clear the toxins and the resulting symptoms.

★ Snot Blend ★

Rub this blend onto your child's chest. For kids over the age of twelve, double the drops of essential oils. To use in a vaporiser, use the same amount of essential oils without the base oil.

- ★ 2 drops German Chamomile

- ★ 2 drops Eucalyptus

- ★ 2 drops Lemon

- ★ 3 drops Peppermint

- ★ 50ml Apricot Kernel oil

Chicken Pox

This contagious, viral infection can only be caught by being in direct contact with someone who has the chicken pox or shingles. Like all viral infections, the state of a person's immune system can determine how the virus runs. It can affect children of any age and can be caught two or three times during childhood. Before the rash and blisters appear, the child can present with mild fever, headache, chills and be just plain cranky. The itch that can come with the rash can be irresistible to scratch but it is important not to because nasty, infected sores can result and lead to scarring. I remember as a kid having socks put on my hands to stop me from scratching!

★ Anti-itch Lotion ★

- ★ 5 drops German Chamomile
- ★ 15 drops Lavender
- ★ 100ml Unscented Body Lotion base

★ Anti-itch Bath Salts ★

- ★ 2 drops Lavender
- ★ 1 drop Tea Tree
- ★ 1 tablespoon unrefined mineral sea salt

Chilblains

Incredibly sore, numb and itchy, chilblains are caused by reduced circulation and a lack of oxygen to an area of the body. They usually appear on extremities such as the hands and feet – I have even had them on my ears. I have experienced them from moving suddenly from hot to cold environments, such as when going from the very cold outside to a nice snuggly heated room inside during winter. Prevention is the key, and the way to prevent chilblains is to improve the circulation to the at risk areas. Essential oils such as Black Pepper, Rosemary, Cypress, Juniper and Geranium are all effective.

★ Chilblains Oil ★

Massage the following blend into vulnerable areas twice daily to prevent or relieve symptoms.

- ★ 4 drops Geranium

- ★ 3 drops Black Pepper

- ★ 3 drops Rosemary

- ★ 4 drops German Chamomile

- ★ 50ml Apricot Kernel oil

Cold Sores

Herpes simplex generally occurs when you are physically or emotionally run down or simply stressed out. From a naturopathic point of view, you have to look at your nutrition and get back on track. Aromatherapy is excellent for treating the external lesion. Cold sores are extremely contagious so treat with care. Some people say that they can feel the tingle before the blister appears, so the sooner you can apply the oil, the better.

★ Cold Sore Dab ★

With a clean cotton bud apply one drop of the essential oil neat onto the lesion.

★ 1 drop Tea Tree

or

★ 1 drop Geranium

or

★ 1 drop Bergamot

If the cold sore is close to the corner of the mouth, I prefer to use Geranium because Tea Tree can sometimes dry out the corners of the mouth too much.

Colds and Flu

Symptoms of colds and flu can vary between children. Whether it is present in their head or chest, look at the child's diet and eliminate dairy and wheat for a few weeks to lessen the production of mucous. Refer to the recipes for catarrh, coughs and fevers as these can all assist, depending on the particular symptoms. Warm baths help to sweat out some toxins and can relieve the aches. Try the following combination in a warm bath or combine with a base oil to make a massage blend.

★ Flu Bath ★

Have your child soak in this bath to help relieve the symptoms of colds and flu.

- ★ 3 drops Tea Tree

- ★ 3 drops Lavender

- ★ 4 drops Ginger

- ★ 50ml dispersing bath oil or 50 g of Epsom Salts

Coughs

Coughs can be the resulting symptoms of asthma or bronchitis or the body simply trying to eliminate a blockage. Whatever the cause, we do not want to suppress the cough, but we do want to relax the breathing and assist in the elimination of the blockage. If the cough is due to a build-up of mucous, essential oil blends such as the recipe recommended for catarrh, combined with Cypress to regulate breathing, are effective.

★ Cough Chest Rub ★

Rub this blend onto your child's chest and throat. For kids over the age of twelve, double the drops of essential oils. To use in a vaporiser, use the same amount of essential oils, without the base oil.

- ★ 2 drops Cypress

- ★ 2 drops Cedarwood

- ★ 2 drops Eucalyptus

- ★ 3 drops Frankincense

- ★ 1 drop Peppermint

- ★ 50ml Apricot Kernel oil

Whooping Cough

This is no ordinary cough, it is a contagious disease that causes the airways to become blocked with mucous. The blockage gives the cough a high-pitched 'whoop' sound, quite unlike a normal cough. It generally starts with cold-like symptoms and turns nasty with the cough escalating after the first week or so. See your medical practitioner if you suspect whooping cough. It can be very draining, so keep the child rested and keep simple foods and water up to prevent dehydration. To treat with aromatherapy, blend the following recipes for a chest rub and for a vaporiser or humidifier. A humid environment helps to loosen the mucous and phlegm, which has to come out in order for the child to recover quickly.

★ Chest Rub ★

- ★ 2 drops Thyme
- ★ 4 drops Frankincense
- ★ 4 drops Myrrh
- ★ 5 drops Tea Tree
- ★ 50ml Apricot Kernel oil

★ Vaporiser / Humidifier Blend ★

- ★ 3 drops Thyme
- ★ 3 drops Eucalyptus
- ★ 2 drops Myrrh
- ★ 2 drops Cypress

Cradle Cap

Cradle cap is the greasy, crusty patches that form on a baby's scalp when there is an over activity of the sebaceous glands and excess sebum is produced. You should never try to pick off the crusty scabs; the crusts need to be softened and the hair needs to be brushed gently. It can take a few weeks to clear.

★ Cradle Cap Scalp Oil ★

Blend the following to create a scalp oil, massage in gently, leave for a few minutes and then shampoo out.

- ★ 2 drops Geranium
- ★ 1 drop Lavender
- ★ 1 drop Tea Tree
- ★ 15ml Avocado oil
- ★ 15ml Jojoba oil
- ★ 20ml Apricot Kernel oil

Croup

The barking sound of a croup cough is heard when there is an infection of the airways, generally it is viral. The upper part of the airways become swollen, which restricts the passage of air and creates the barking sound. It mainly occurs in young children under the age of three. Symptoms are usually exacerbated by the cool, dry night air. Treatment involves increasing the humidity of the room. The only real way to get enough steam is to run the bath or shower and close off the bathroom. By adding essential oils to the bath you are effectively sitting in a room that is one giant vaporiser.

★ Chest Rub ★

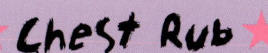

Rub over chest and throat. To use in a vaporiser, blend the same essential oils without the base oil.

★ 1 drop Eucalyptus

★ 1 drop Thyme

★ 1 drop German Chamomile

★ 2 drops Cypress

★ 50ml Apricot Kernel oil

83

Cuts and Scratches

It's inevitable – kids are going to experience cuts and scratches. Most will be minor and will be able to be treated at home. Please use common sense, if a wound is deep, see the doctor to get it treated. Most kids will end up having stitches at some time during their younger years. And after all the tears and emotions are over, these experiences make great stories to be shared at school. Treating cuts and scratches is easy.

★ Cuts and Scratches First Aid ★

- ★ First, apply gentle pressure to stop any bleeding.

- ★ Bathe the area with 2 drops of Tea Tree oil diluted in approximately 1 cup of water.

- ★ Place 1 drop each of Lavender and Tea Tree on a sterile dressing and when the oils dry, apply the dressing to the wound.

- ★ Change the dressing and oils daily until healed.

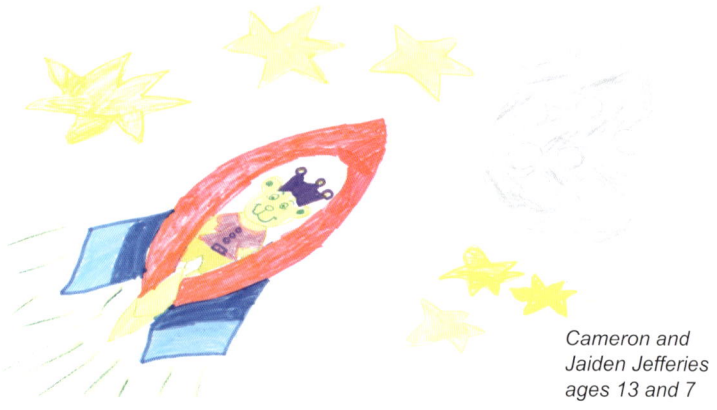

Cameron and Jaiden Jefferies ages 13 and 7

Dandruff

Psoriasis or eczema on the scalp can be confused with dandruff and naturopathically we treat these conditions in a similar way. Many people use anti-dandruff shampoos and treatments, which contain some pretty interesting chemicals that I'd prefer to not see used on any person. The natural alternative is to use a Rosemary-based shampoo and scalp oil to rectify the imbalance.

★ Scalp Oil ★

Dampen the hair, apply a small amount of scalp oil (about the size of a twenty-cent piece), massage into the scalp, leave in overnight (place an old towel on the pillow to minimise any oil residue) and wash out with a Rosemary shampoo in the morning.

★ 2 drops Rosemary

★ 4 drops Geranium

★ 2 drops Tea Tree

★ 2 drops Cedarwood

★ 10ml Carrot infused oil

★ 10ml Jojoba oil

★ 10ml Avocado oil

★ 20ml Rosehip oil

85

Deodorant

As kids start becoming teenagers and their hormones kick in, body odour can start to occur. There are no essential oils that will stop perspiration, we all need to sweat, but you can use them to reduce body odour effectively.

★ Deodorant ★

Use in a 100ml spray bottle

- ★ 4 drops Tea Tree

- ★ 8 drops Geranium

- ★ 8 drops Patchouli

- ★ 4 drops Cypress

- ★ 24 drops Essential Oil Soluboliser

- ★ 90ml filtered water

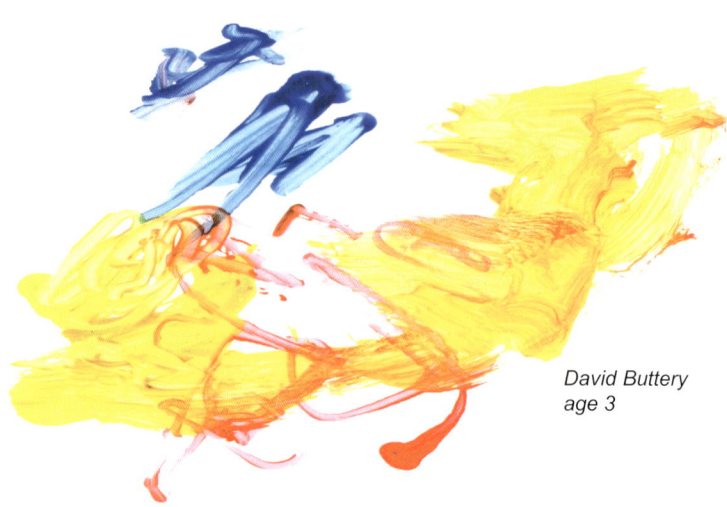

David Buttery
age 3

Deodorocks

I really like 'The Rock' (also known as kaolinite) which is a naturally occurring mineral that has been used for centuries by cultures such as the Egyptians and Chinese. It's main component is potash crystal and it also contains calcium, magnesium, potassium and sodium. It occurs as a clay mineral formed by the weathering or hydrothermal alteration of feldspars or aluminous silicates. The deodorock has many uses, the most popular as an underarm deodorant, but it may also be used as a foot deodorant. It works by leaving a fine layer of dissolved minerals on the surface of the skin, which inhibits the growth of odour-causing bacteria. The deodorock is not an anti-perspirant, it allows you to still perspire but without the smell.

Advantages of the deodorock over conventional deodorant:

★ Free from harmful aluminum sulphate.

★ Has no scent of its own to clash with your perfume.

★ Does not stain clothes.

★ Does not spill or leak— especially beneficial when travelling.

★ Contains no artificial additives or ozone depleting chemicals.

★ Can be used on all skin types.

★ Lasts up to twelve or eighteen months.

How do you use it?

After showering, simply wet the rock with water and apply by gently rubbing onto the underarms or the soles of the feet. After use, rinse and dry off with a towel. If you drop the rock and it breaks, pick up the pieces and place in a spray bottle filled with purified water. The rock will dissolve and you can use it as a spray-on deodorant. Deodorocks are available from health food or natural therapies stores.

Digestion

Colic

A build-up of gas in the digestive system is a very painful experience for a baby and is distressing for the parents who are trying to relieve him or her. Colic can result from a number of causes, including the food and drink the breast-feeding mother is consuming throughout the day or if baby eats too quickly. The pain subsides when a burp or bowel motion releases the trapped gas. Some preventatives that I have found useful include having the breastfeeding mother drink fennel seed herbal tea and the use of a warm compress, made with Fennel essential oil, applied to the breast. The antispasmodic benefits of Fennel pass through to the mother's milk helping to settle the baby and prevent a build-up of gas.

★ Tummy Colic Massage Oil ★

Rub on baby's tummy gently in a clockwise direction.

★   3 drops Fennel

★   2 drops Mandarin

★   2 drops Tangerine

★   2 drops German Chamomile

★   50ml Apricot Kernel oil

Constipation

Technically, constipation is not just the absence of stools, but also when a person is passing little pebbly poos. It can be caused by many factors including an unbalanced diet, dehydration and emotional stress. When kids are being toilet trained they can hang on for very long periods of time because of the emotional stress of it all. It's important to make them feel as comfortable as possible and to make the potty experience a relaxed one. If they hang on for too long the stool can become dry and painful to pass, which can lead to a negative memory association and exacerbate the problem.

How do you treat constipation? First, look at the child's water intake and recent health – dehydration is the most common cause of constipation in both children and adults, followed by a lack of fibre in the diet, even a fever can cause dehydration which can lead to constipation. If the child is dehydrated, the motion will literally be too dry to move easily. The bowel runs in a clockwise direction and a simple tummy massage is part of an effective treatment. A firm but gentle pressure is required, if the child has been constipated for a while the tummy will be tender. If constipation lasts longer than one week see a medical practitioner.

★ Constipation Tummy Oil ★

Rub this blend onto your child's tummy in a clockwise direction.

- ★ 1 drop Mandarin
- ★ 2 drops Marjoram
- ★ 1 drop Orange
- ★ 1 drop Rosemary
- ★ 50ml Apricot Kernel oil

Diarrhoea

More serious than constipation, diarrhoea can cause dehydration very quickly in a small child. It should not go unchecked for more than 24 hours. Loose stools are not diarrhoea. Diarrhoea is when the stool becomes abnormally frequent and watery for that particular person. In children, teething, colds, food sensitivity, earaches, stress and viral or bacterial stomach infections can all cause diarrhoea. Diarrhoea is the body trying to clear toxins and it will naturally run its course. A treatment plan includes reducing solid foods, maintaining fluid intake and drinking an electrolyte solution, which you can buy from the chemist. Tummy rubs can also ease the symptoms, blend the following combination and use as required massaging with a firm but gentle pressure.

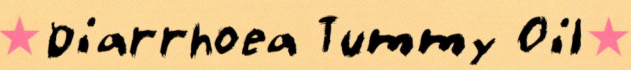

★Diarrhoea Tummy Oil★

Rub this blend onto your child's tummy in a clockwise direction.

- ★ 2 drops German Chamomile

- ★ 2 drops Neroli

- ★ 3 drops Lavender

- ★ 2 drops Tea Tree

- ★ 50ml Apricot Kernel oil

Earache

Colds, tonsillitis, teething, bacterial or viral infections such as mumps can all be causes behind an earache. The pain can be tremendous and can radiate down the neck. Try to identify the cause and see a medical practitioner if required. I remember when I was a kid, if we had an earache, Mum would warm up some olive oil and put a few drops into the ear and seal with a cotton wool plug. Nowadays, I prefer you to use Jojoba oil as a base because it is a liquid wax.

★ Earache Oil ★

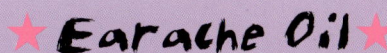

Blend the following recipe and use to massage around the ear, surrounding jaw line and neck. Then place a few drops into the ear and gently seal with a cotton wool plug. Ensure the plug is not too small and that you do not push it far inside the ear.

★ 3 drops German Chamomile

★ 3 drops Lavender

★ 2 drops Thyme

★ 50ml Jojoba oil

Fever

Fever is the body reacting to a viral or bacterial infection, measles, mumps, chickenpox, teething, tonsillitis and so on. It is a good sign that the body is working and fighting something. If a child were unwell and had no fever, I might be worried. The shivers are a symptom of the body trying to cool its core temperature. Fevers need to be addressed and closely monitored, watch for dehydration and give lukewarm sponge baths regularly using the following blend of essential oils. You can also use this blend to make a cool water compress for the body and forehead.

★ **Fever Sponge Bath** ★

Sponge over forehead, arms and legs.

- ★ 2 drops Spearmint

- ★ 3 drops Lavender

- ★ 3 drops German Chamomile

- ★ 2 drops Eucalyptus

- ★ 50ml dispersing bath oil

Gingivitis and Bleeding Gums

Bleeding gums can be caused by poor oral hygiene and/or a vitamin C deficiency. To maintain good oral hygiene, make a mouthwash from 5 drops of Myrrh Tincture in warm water. Use after brushing the teeth, swish around and spit out.

If the gums are bleeding and there are no signs of gingivitis, look at your vitamin C levels. One of the first signs of scurvy is bleeding gums, people don't think of scurvy nowadays, but it is still around. If experiencing bleeding gums, take a vitamin C supplement as well as using the Myrrh Tincture mouthwash.

Glands – Swollen

Swollen lymph glands are a good sign because it shows that the body is fighting an infection and that the glands are doing what they are designed to do. The lymphatic system filters your blood and the lymph glands are like little dams where the toxins collect. The infection could be viral or bacterial, either way we treat it in the same way with compresses. It is also wise to see your naturopath for a herbal tincture for internal treatment and always take vitamin C.

★ Swollen Glands Massage Oil ★

Massage around the affected area or put 10 drops into a bowl of warm to hot water and use as a compress.

- ★ 4 drops Tea Tree

- ★ 4 drops Thyme

- ★ 6 drops German Chamomile

- ★ 50ml Apricot Kernel oil

93

Growing Pains

This is a recipe for older kiddies who may be experiencing growing pains or who are starting to play more vigorous sports. For use with sports-related aches and pains, blend a combination containing more stimulating and antispasmodic oils such as Black Pepper which will be good for relieving aches and warming the muscles before exercise.

★ Growing Pain Massage Oil ★

Massage over area that is hurting. For children over the age of ten, increase the strength by doubling the drops of essential oils

★ 1 drop German Chamomile

★ 2 drops Marjoram

★ 2 drops Lavender

★ 10ml Hypericum infused oil

★ 40ml Sweet Almond oil

Hay fever

Antigens such as dust, pollens, powders and insecticides can grab sensitive people and cause symptoms such as a runny nose, sneezing, and itchy, watery eyes. Whatever the cause, the symptoms need to be relieved. When you know what it is that the child is sensitive to, make an effort to keep them away from the triggers and work on their immune system to reduce their sensitivity.

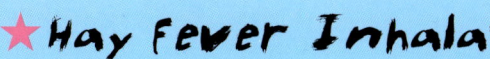

★ Hay Fever Inhalation ★

Place this blend in a vaporiser, inhale using a bowl of warm water, or place on a handkerchief.

- ★ 2 drops German Chamomile

- ★ 1 drop Eucalyptus

- ★ 2 drops Pine

- ★ 3 drops Lavender

- ★ 2 drops Lemon

- ★ 2 drops Peppermint

Headaches

Most headaches are a result of either stress or dehydration, but there can be other causes too such as eyestrain, lack of sleep, teething, stomach ache and head colds. Headaches can also be a sign of something more serious, if they persist check with your naturopath or medical practitioner. How do you treat a headache? First, make sure that the child is not dehydrated; give him or her a glass of water. Then, I like to use a cool compress on the forehead and back of the neck.

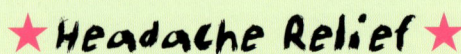

★ Headache Relief ★

★ Blend 2 drops each of Lavender and Spearmint into a bowl of cool water.

★ Dip a flannel into the water and place it on the forehead and back of the neck.

★ Refresh the flannel as the coolness subsides and repeat as needed.

★ Have the child rest until the headache passes; if they continue to race around the treatment will not be as effective.

Head Lice

As soon as school starts, so too do the lice. Lice are no fun for anyone – not the kids nor Mum and Dad who have to keep cleaning their heads. One of the most effective remedies I have found is to make a scalp oil using the following blend.

★ Head Lice Scalp Oil ★

- ★ 3 drops Rosemary

- ★ 2 drops Patchouli

- ★ 1 drop Ylang Ylang

- ★ 4 drops Tea Tree

- ★ 50ml Jojoba oil

Instructions:

1. Dampen the hair; massage the oil into the scalp and hair and leave in overnight (put an old towel on the pillow, so the oil doesn't go everywhere).

2. Shampoo out the next morning.

3. Follow up with one of those little lice combs to remove the dead bodies and any eggs.

The scalp oil is effective in killing the lice and eggs. It leaves the hair very soft which makes it difficult for the lice to re-attach. After the initial treatment to remove the critters, you can make up the following preventative recipe.

★ Preventative Lice Spray ★

Add the essential oils to the soluboliser in a spray bottle, top up with water and shake well. Spray and brush through dry hair each day.

- ★ 5 drops Tea Tree

- ★ 5 drops Eucalyptus

- ★ 10 drops Rosemary

- ★ 30 drops Essential Oil Soluboliser

Heat Rash (prickly heat)

Heat rash is a temporary skin eruption caused by excess sweating and over heating. It is seen more on babies because their sweat glands may not have matured enough to cope with the hot weather. Prickly heat is a collection of tiny red blister-like bumps in a rash formation that can be insanely itchy. Treatment includes pulling the excess heat out of the skin and settling the rash. Use the following blend in a lukewarm bath. When the child is taken out of the bath, pat them dry remembering not to rub too vigorously.

★ Soothing Bath Oil ★

- ★ 1 drop Eucalyptus

- ★ 1 drop Spearmint

- ★ 8 drops Lavender

- ★ 50ml dispersing bath oil

Hives — Urticaria

I have many memories of experiencing hives throughout my life, I remember once as a kid at the local football club, having my whole face swell like one giant hive. Even on a recent trip to New Zealand, after indulging in too many thermal hot spring baths (rich in sulphur), my lips blew up in one giant hive. It was hilarious going through customs to fly back to Australia later that day! Yes, we can all still experience some imbalances, even when we're grown ups.

Hives are raised white or red inflamed, irritated and incredibly itchy skin reactions, and the more you scratch the worse they get. They can come from allergies to plants in the garden, medications or as a result of another infection. The bottom line is that they are distressing to the person who has them and to those who have to see them. Aromatherapy treatment involves compresses, massages or baths. Vitamin C is excellent for at reducing the allergic itch and will help to reduce the swelling faster.

★ Hives Massage Oil ★

For older children, double the drops of essential oils. To make a compress, use the same essential oils without the base oil. To make a bath oil, supplement the Jojoba oil for dispersing bath oil.

- ★ 4 drops German Chamomile

- ★ 4 drops Lavender

- ★ 2 drops Spearmint

- ★ 50ml Jojoba oil

Impetigo

Also known as 'school sores', this is an extremely contagious skin infection presenting as pus-filled sores. The sores generally appear on the face first but can spread anywhere. I remember Mum telling us as kids not to walk through the long grass because if a child had school sores and had walked through earlier, we could catch them. Mums are always right. Because it is so contagious, you need to be careful when treating impetigo and always use disposable cloths/swabs. To bathe, place 10 drops of Tea Tree and 10 drops of Lavender into a bowl containing approximately 100ml of warm water. Also blend the following to create an oil that can be applied directly to the sore to promote healing.

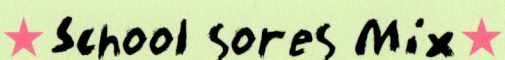

★ School Sores Mix ★

Apply directly to the sore.

★ 4 drops Lavender

★ 4 drops German Chamomile

★ 2 drops Tea Tree

★ 2 drops Thyme

★ 50ml Calendula infused oil

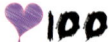

Insomnia

Little brains go fast, so how do we switch them off at night? The first thing to do is prepare the environment for sleep, if the whole household is busy at night you cannot expect a child to just switch off on demand. Remember, kids pick up on your energy, if you are being 'go-fast', they will too.

Use relaxing essential oils throughout the evening to slow everyone down to a relaxed pace. Try the following blend in your oil vaporiser and enjoy the relaxing effects. With small children, blend the grounding bath oil and watch them slow down. This recipe can also be made into a massage oil, using Apricot Kernel as the carrier oil.

★ Sleep Easy Vaporiser Blend ★

Use this blend to slow everyone down to a relaxed pace.

- ★ 2 drops German Chamomile
- ★ 2 drops Cedarwood
- ★ 5 drops Lime
- ★ 3 drops Petitgrain

★ Grounding Bath Oil ★

- ★ 8 drops Lavender
- ★ 5 drops Mandarin
- ★ 1 drop Vetiver
- ★ 50ml dispersing bath oil

Menstrual problems - teenagers

For the reproductive system to be whole and functioning in a well-balanced way the body, mind and spirit must all be well and thriving. Your context (everything influencing your internal and external emotional and physical health) needs to be balanced; imbalances in any one area can be a cause behind reproductive system imbalances and the symptoms that go along with them. Think about what is happening in your world, and see where you can restore some balance. In clinic I found it common for teenagers to be living out of balance.

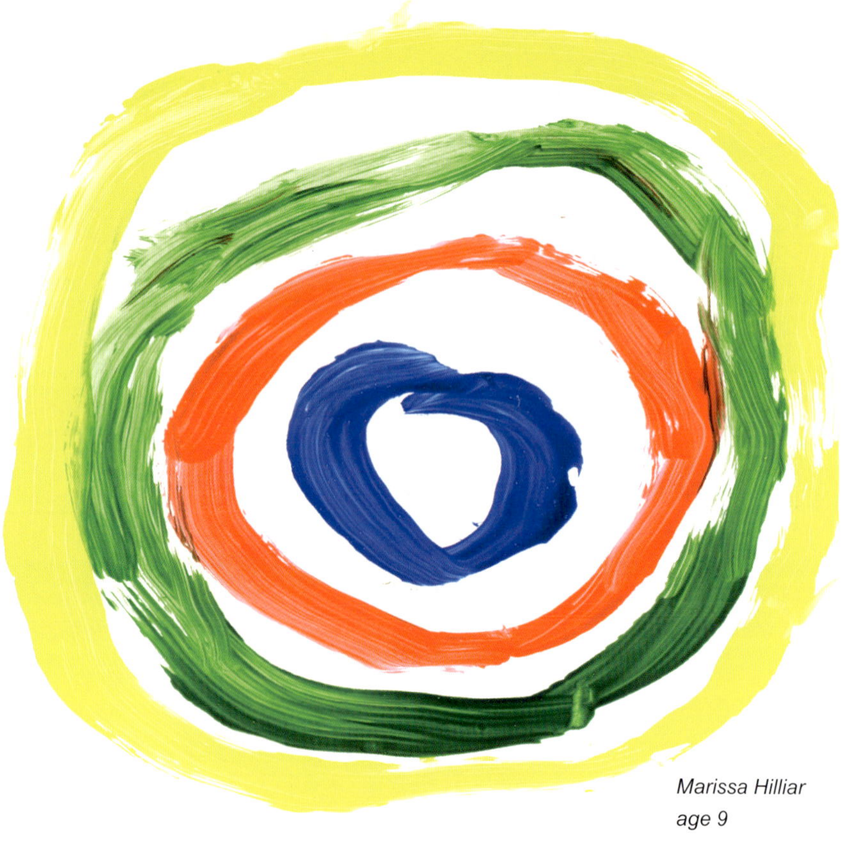

Marissa Hilliar
age 9

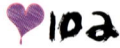

PMT

Pre-menstrual tension occurs through an imbalance of oestrogen and progesterone levels in the body, which occurs just before the period and can create a roller coaster of emotions that can be difficult to understand for the person experiencing it. It can be difficult enough as an adult, let alone for a teenager. Apart from the mood swings, some women experience bloating, swollen breasts and more. In my experience the symptoms generally settle down once the period begins. The following is a basic blend that I have used successfully with teenagers. All women are individuals and will present with their own symptoms, see your aromatherapist or naturopath if you require something more specific for your symptoms.

★ PMT Tummy Rub ★

Massage over the abdomen twice daily from mid-cycle until the period begins. Apply in a clockwise, circular motion.

- ★ 5 drops Fennel

- ★ 6 drops Geranium

- ★ 6 drops Bergamot

- ★ 4 drops Rosewood

- ★ 4 drops Neroli

- ★ 50ml Evening Primrose oil

103

Amenorrhoea
– absence of menstruation

For young girls, menstruation can be scant for the first year or so. It can also be delayed or can start and then go away again. Factors that usually create this imbalance are emotional or physical stresses. Aromatherapy can help to rectify the problem, but if it persists visit your naturopath to get a herbal tincture to complement the aromatherapy treatment.

 Amenorrhoea Tummy Rub

Massage on tummy twice daily.

★ 4 drops Clary Sage

★ 6 drops Cypress

★ 8 drops Geranium

★ 4 drops Fennel

★ 50ml Evening Primrose oil

Dysmenorrhoea
– painful difficult periods

Blend the following to help relieve muscle spasms and cramps. You can also use these same essential oils to create a compress or blend into a dispersing bath oil base to create a wonderful body soak. Please also see your naturopath for additional nutritional and herbal remedies.

★ Menstrual Pain Massage Oil ★

Massage into the tummy or back area (where the pain is) as required.

- ★ 4 drops Clary Sage

- ★ 6 drops Peppermint

- ★ 4 drops Cypress

- ★ 2 drops Rose

- ★ 5 drops Lavender

- ★ 4 drops Black Pepper

- ★ 50ml Evening Primrose oil

Nappy Rash

Being in a wet and warm nappy for too long is generally what causes this skin condition. Nappy rash can also be aggravated by sensitivities to chemical cleaning solutions and products. Either way, it is a painful rash that can become infected and progress to become sores and even pustules. Nappy rash must be treated promptly. Blend the following to make a body oil for the affected area. Also use these same essential oils with essential oil souboliser for use in the bath. Let the baby's bottom be nappy and pants free for some time each day, the cool and dry fresh air will help the healing process, and if possible, let their bottom see a little sunshine too.

★ Bottom Soother ★

- ★ 2 drops German Chamomile
- ★ 2 drops Lavender
- ★ 1 drop Tea Tree
- ★ 25ml Jojoba oil
- ★ 25ml Calendula oil

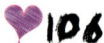

Ringworm

Ringworm presents as a red ring-shaped fungal rash with a clear centre. It can be extremely itchy and is contagious, so be careful with washing and sharing clothes. In my clinic I have used an old remedy on children over ten years of age, in which I cut a raw clove of garlic and rub it directly onto the ringworm. Make sure that you do not get it on the good skin around the ringworm. It is very effective but cannot be used on small children. With children under the age of ten, use the following recipe; it will also help to take the itch out of the skin.

★ Ringworm Oil ★

Apply with a cotton bud to the affected area.

- ★ 4 drops Lavender
- ★ 2 drops Geranium
- ★ 4 drops Patchouli
- ★ 4 drops Tea Tree
- ★ 25ml Calendula oil
- ★ 25ml Jojoba oil

Scars

Kids are going to knock themselves around a bit and get the odd set of stitches. Once the initial hurt has healed and after the stitches have been removed, apply the following blend. The sooner you begin treating a scar, the faster it will reduce. Rosehip oil is rich in omega-3 and omega-6 essential fatty acids making it the perfect base for reducing the chances of permanent scarring.

★ Scar Healing Oil ★

Apply twice daily to the affected area, providing that there is no broken skin. If the skin is broken, you must wait until it has healed before applying this blend.

- ★ 6 drops Frankincense

- ★ 4 drops Neroli

- ★ 8 drops Lavender

- ★ 50ml Rosehip oil

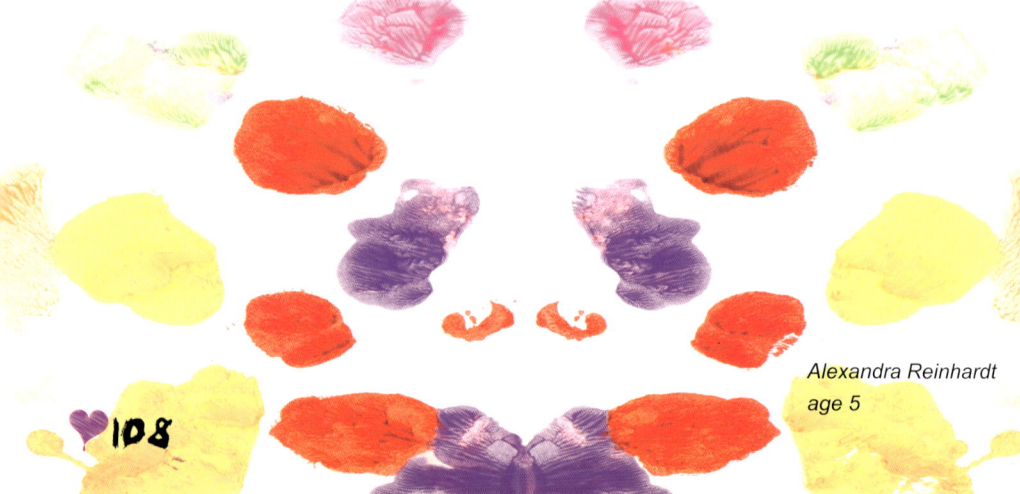

Alexandra Reinhardt
age 5

Sinusitis

This is the bacterial infection that comes from inefficient drainage of nasal mucous and commonly runs with or after colds and flu or hay fever. Symptoms can include headache and toothache, loss of smell, tenderness over the face and a pressure build-up in the head. Use a chest rub over the neck and chest and also use these same essential oils in a bowl of hot water as an inhalation; the steam assists in loosening the mucous. A warm compress on the cheeks and forehead with the same oil blend will also assist mucous movement.

★ Chest Rub ★

For kids over the age of twelve, double the amount of essential oils. To use in a vaporiser, use the same essential oils without the base oil.

- ★ 3 drops Ginger

- ★ 3 drops Myrrh

- ★ 2 drops Thyme

- ★ 2 drops Pine

- ★ 2 drops Frankincense

- ★ 4 drops Peppermint

- ★ 50ml Apricot Kernel oil

Skin Ailments

Eczema and Dermatitis

Eczema and dermatitis can occur as a result of allergies or sensitivities to foods, chemicals and many other things in life. Whatever the aggravating agent is, contact with it must be avoided to assist the healing process. For example, if the condition is being caused by a sensitivity to dairy products, eliminate them from the diet immediately (dairy products and refined foods are a common cause of these two skin conditions. Seek advice from your naturopath before eliminating any foods from a child's diet.) The symptoms of eczema and dermatitis can range from dry and scaly, to red and inflamed skin, use the appropriate blend to create a massage oil and apply as required to relieve the symptoms.

★ Dry and Scaly ★

- ★ 2 drops Frankincense

- ★ 2 drops Rose

- ★ 2 drops Palmarosa

- ★ 3 drops German Chamomile

- ★ 3 drops Lavender

- ★ 20ml Jojoba oil

- ★ 15ml Evening Primrose oil

- ★ 15ml Rosehip oil

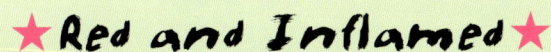

★ Red and Inflamed ★

- ★ 5 drops German Chamomile

- ★ 4 drops Lavender

- ★ 4 drops Neroli

- ★ 10ml Rosehip oil

- ★ 40ml Jojoba oil

Psoriasis

Psoriasis can be caused by many factors, both physical and emotional. The look of the skin will vary from person to person, as will the way it spreads. I have treated many people over the years with this condition including some adults and children who have been covered from head to toe with psoriasis. The emotional stress over the discomfort and appearance can exacerbate the symptoms.

Use essential oils for relaxation first, and then blend the following recipes to treat the symptoms. I have had great success with these but if you wish to have something made specifically for yourself or your child consult your aromatherapist or naturopath. As with eczema and dermatitis, diet plays a part as well, consult your naturopath for advice as to how your diet might be affecting you. Use the eczema and dermatitis recipes above to treat the symptoms.

Acne and the Teenager's Skin

The skin is simply a reflection of what is happening on the inside of the body. Hormones start churning around the teenage years and one of the most noticeable changes your child will experience is in their skin. Most acne products on the market contain alcohols, which dry out pimples, but cause the body to think that the skin in that particular area is dry – so it responds by increasing the output of oils. This creates the typical dry/oily cycle. There are number of essential oils that will help to balance the hormones and oil production in the skin. Also, remember to look at your teenager's nutrition.

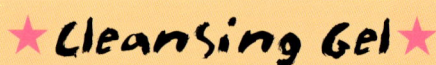 ★ **Cleansing Gel** ★

Blend the following combination of antiseptic and detoxifying essential oils to rebalance the skin's oil production.

- ★ 8 drops Geranium

- ★ 4 drops Juniper

- ★ 6 drops Lavender

- ★ 2 drops Tea Tree

- ★ 100ml Unscented natural shower gel base

★ Moisturising Cream ★

Use for confused teenage skin that's oily one day and dry the next to balance the classic oily T-zone.

- ★ 8 drops Geranium

- ★ 4 drops Juniper

- ★ 6 drops Lavender

- ★ 2 drops Tea Tree

- ★ 100grams Unscented vegetable cream base or Jojoba oil

★ Balancing/Moisturising Gel ★

Combine the following blend of essential oils to help soothe and moisturise a teenager's angry skin.

- ★ 10 drops Lavender

- ★ 6 drops Geranium

- ★ 4 drops Juniper

- ★ 100ml pure aloe vera gel

Sore Throat/ Strep Throat

This can result from anything that is irritating the sensitive mucous membranes at the back of the throat, including cigarette smoke, dust, fumes as well as infections, abrasions and chronic coughing.

A teaspoon of unrefined pure honey from the health food shop sucked slowly will help to settle the symptoms, combine this with the use of an aromatherapy chest/throat rub.

★ Sore Throat Rub ★

Rub over the chest and throat. For kids over the age of twelve, double the drops of essential oils. To use in a vaporiser, use the same essential oils without the base oil.

- ★ 5 drops Lemon

- ★ 2 drops Ginger

- ★ 6 drops Sandalwood

- ★ 4 drops Frankincense

- ★ 4 drops Tea Tree

- ★ 50ml Apricot Kernel oil

Sprains and Strains

Ligaments and muscles can wear the brunt of childhood games and play. A child does not have to be competing in a sport to experience a sprain or strain. I was constantly spraining my ankles as a child, I remember doing it one time on the way home from school. Once you have gone over on an ankle it can take a long while to heal and the injury gets aggravated again easily. As with any soft tissue injury, follow the usual first aid protocol of 'Rest, Ice, Compression and Elevation'. Use common sense; if you think the injury needs an x-ray see your medical practitioner.

In the first instance, make a cold compress with 5 drops of Lavender, 3 drops of Spearmint and 5 drops of German Chamomile in 200ml of cold water. Soak a flannel in the solution and place on the injured area. Re-dip the flannel as it begins to lose its coolness. Once the heat has left the injured site, usually after forty-eight hours, you can start to use heat to break-up and draw out the bruising. Blend the following essential oils and use twice daily until healed.

★ Sprain Massage Oil ★

- ★ 5 drops Black Pepper
- ★ 5 drops Rosemary
- ★ 4 drops Ginger
- ★ 4 drops Marjoram
- ★ 50ml Arnica infused oil

Stress

This is a modern, overused word for 'life'. We all get 'wound-up' sometimes but it is sad to see increasing numbers of kids feeling that way too. I don't think kids get the chance to be kids long enough these days, it's as though they know too much and take on worries that they shouldn't have to.

Using aromatherapy essential oils around your home can help enormously to balance life out. Try one of these simple vaporiser blends.

★ Chill Out Blend ★

- ★ 2 drops Clary Sage
- ★ 2 drops German Chamomile
- ★ 1 drop Cedarwood
- ★ 4 drops Lime
- ★ 2 drops Petitgrain

★ Settle Petal Blend ★

- ★ 3 drops Mandarin
- ★ 4 drops Orange
- ★ 4 drops Lime
- ★ 5 drops Lavender

Study

I was never one for wanting to do my homework and, like most adults, I wish I had applied myself more at school! But there were always so many more fun things to do other than study. Use this blend in your vaporiser to help stop procrastination and ground the child so that they can sit still and get their homework done. This works for big people too. Because our memories are so closely linked to our sense of smell, if you use your study blend regularly and then take it with you into exams, the memory association will help you to recall information more easily. Just put a drop of your study blend onto your collar or a tissue and inhale.

★ Focus Blend ★

Increase concentration and focus by using these essential oils in a vaporiser or on a tissue to inhale.

- ★ 3 drops Peppermint

- ★ 2 drops Rosemary

- ★ 3 drops Lemon

- ★ 2 drops Ginger

- ★ 1 drop Vetiver

 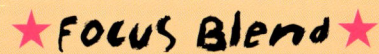

Styes

Remember the old remedy of rubbing the gold wedding ring on the stye? A stye is a bacterial infection on the edge of the upper or lower eyelid. It can vary in size from a small pimple-like swelling to an all-out infection which almost closes the eye. Styes can spread and need to be treated very carefully. Because eyes are so sensitive, we do not recommend that you use essential oils in that area. The treatment I have used with clients in the past involves chamomile tea. Chamomile is a wonderful anti-inflammatory, which will take the angriness out of the stye and bring the pus to a head. Do not squeeze the stye. Continue using the chamomile tea until it has cleared.

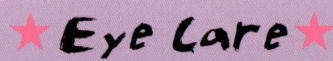

★ Eye Care ★

- ★ Make a cup of chamomile tea; allow it to cool to a temperature that you can place on your eye area.

- ★ Use a clean cotton pad and soak it in the tea, then ring it out enough to use.

- ★ Place it over the eye and rest for five minutes.

- ★ Repeat three times a day until healed.

Sunburn

As with treating burns, this is a time when we do not add essentials oils to a vegetable oil base, because the vegetable oil will literally cook with the heat that is in the skin, which could promote blistering. The way we treat sunburn is to blend essential oils into a pure Aloe Vera gel base. The Aloe Vera helps in the soothing and healing process.

★ Sunburn Gel ★

Apply as required.

★ 20 drops Lavender

★ 10 drops German Chamomile

★ 10 drops Spearmint

★ 100ml pure Aloe Vera gel

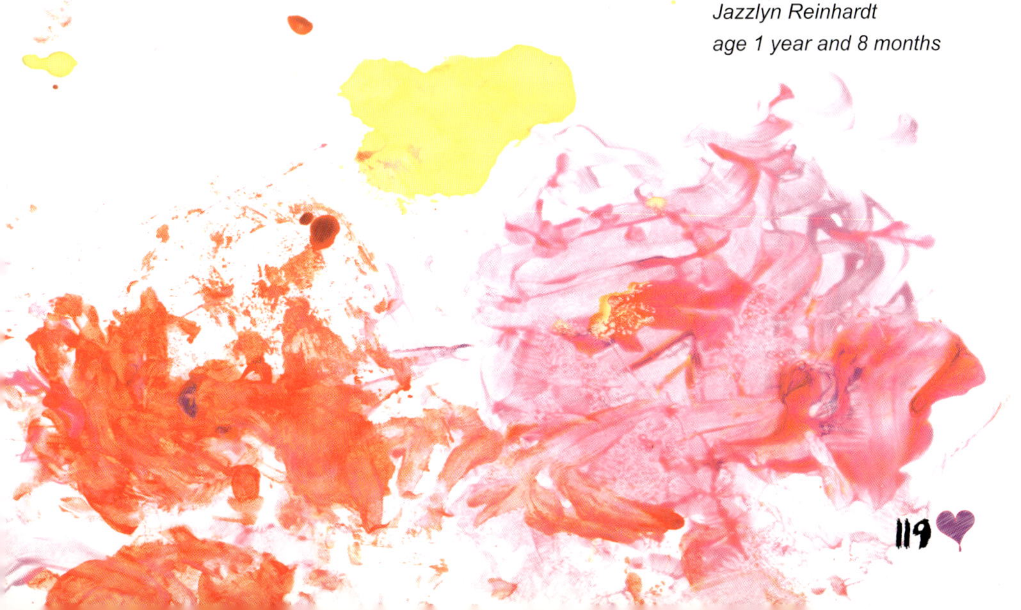

Jazzlyn Reinhardt
age 1 year and 8 months

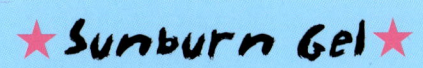

119

Heal their bodies

Teething

Some babies go through the adventures of teething relatively easily but for others it is no fun at all. There is no particular reason why some are okay and others are not. The bottom line is, if you have a child experiencing teething difficulties it can be a pretty miserable time for everyone at home.

They scream because their gums are inflamed and very painful and the regular pharmacy gels and products can tend to not be so effective. We have had great success over the years with a basic aromatherapy oil blend that you rub onto the outside of the baby's cheeks. The anti-inflammatory and soothing properties of the oils bring relief and help to settle the child.

★ Teething Blend ★

Apply this blend to the outside of your child's cheeks as often as required.

★ 3 drops German Chamomile

★ 2 drops Lavender

★ 25ml Jojoba oil

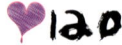120

Toothache

There are many causes of toothache; it may be tooth decay, a mouth injury or infected gums. Whatever the cause, it can be very painful and it generally happens on a weekend or night when you cannot get in to see the dentist. A basic massage oil to apply to the cheeks can work as an anti-inflammatory and analgesic. Combine the following oils and use as required.

★ **Toothache Oil** ★

Apply to the outside of the cheeks.

- ★ 1 drop Clove

- ★ 3 drops German Chamomile

- ★ 2 drops Lavender

- ★ 25ml Jojoba oil

Alexandra Reinhardt age 5

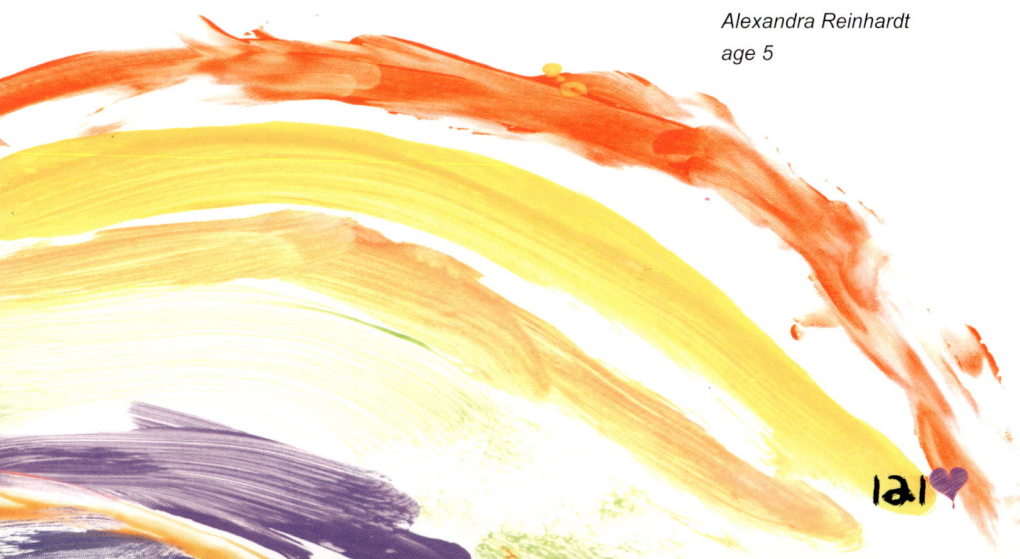

121

Umbilical Cord Infection

The remaining stump of the baby's cord is meant to dry, shrivel up and fall off around seven to ten days after birth. But sometimes the cord can become infected if body excretions have seeped into the area. Mothers are generally advised to use surgical spirit to dry up the cord to assist it in falling off.

In aromatherapy we prefer the use of Lavender oil.

★ Belly Button Bathing Mix ★

★ Place 1 drop of Lavender oil on a cotton bud, and immerse it in warm salty water, squeeze out excess liquid and swab around the cord area.

★ Repeat the treatment with each nappy change. Newborn babies have sensitive skin so just treat the umbilical area.

★ Never try to remove the cord yourself, nature will take its course and it will fall off when it is ready.

★ If the area begins to look inflamed and swollen see your medical practitioner or midwife.

Urinary Tract Infection

Kids of any size can experience a urinary tract infection. The most common urinary infection is cystitis. You cannot play around with urinary system infections; so at the onset of the child complaining or it being painful to pee, check it out. If it hurts to pee, the natural reaction is to stop drinking water, which will only aggravate the problem because the body needs to be flushed of the bacteria that is causing the infection. Keep your child's fluids up with water and cranberry juice, which can be helpful in relieving the burning feeling.

★ Urinary Tract Soothing Oil ★

Massage the back and abdomen regularly.

* ★ 4 drops Tea Tree

* ★ 2 drops Juniper

* ★ 2 drops Bergamot

* ★ 3 drops German Chamomile

* ★ 3 drops Sandalwood

* ★ 50ml Apricot Kernel oil

Viral Diseases

Measles/ German Measles etc

All are contagious, and generally by the time you realise that the child has it, they can be near the end of the contagious period, but it is still important that you keep them isolated and rested. Kids generally pull through easily with no bad side effects, but with the strength of their immune system reduced, they can be susceptible to other infections, so use common sense and care. The initial symptoms can be similar to a cold or flu and include a red, itchy rash that starts as spots inside the mouth and gradually spreads down the body. Treat individual symptoms as they occur and give regular aromatherapy baths to settle the rash. Blend the following oils to use in the bath or as a compress.

★ Viral-goobies Bath Oil ★

- ★ 6 drops Lavender
- ★ 4 drops Tea Tree
- ★ 50ml dispersing bath oil

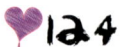

Vomiting

As with diarrhoea, vomiting can lead to dehydration very quickly and so must be monitored carefully. If the child is simply regurgitating their food, it's no big stress, but if the child does the projectile-type vomit, seek advice from a medical practitioner. With young children I have found that the following combination on a tissue to inhale, or used in a compress, helps to settle their stomachs. If you are travelling in a car and motion sickness has got them, use the same essential oils in your car vaporiser both as a preventative before they start feeling sick, as well as to settle their stomachs when they already do. Metaphysically, vomiting is said to be about rejecting new ideas or change, so also consider what might be emotionally distressing the child at the time.

★ Anti-puke Inhalation ★

Place the drops of essential oil on a tissue to inhale or use in a compress.

- ★ 2 drops Spearmint
- ★ 2 drops Lavender

Warts

Kill a toad and bury it at an old cemetery on a full moon to rid your body of warts – sounds pretty cool, but not fun! I have heard so many crazy stories about how to get rid of warts. Aromatherapy is effective; so don't worry about killing toads and so on. Warts are a viral infection that shows up as a benign skin growth that can appear anywhere on the body, but they are generally seen on the hands and legs. They are transmitted by direct contact so it is important that the child does not go picking or playing with them. If they are picked and bleeding or getting red and inflamed, see your medical practitioner. To treat with aromatherapy, combine the following oils and apply a drop of the solution directly to the wart daily until it dries up and falls off. Use care to get the solution only on the wart and not on the surrounding good skin. Cover the wart if the child is tempted to pick at it or play with it.

★ Healing Wart Oil ★

Apply to area daily.

- ★ 15 drops Lemon

- ★ 10 drops Thyme

- ★ 15 drops Bergamot

- ★ 25ml Wheatgerm oil

What Grandmas are made of

as told by a third-grader

A grandmother is a lady who has no children of her own, she likes other peoples' little girls and boys and they love her. A grandfather is a man grandmother. Grandmothers don't have to do anything except be there. They're old so they shouldn't play hard or run. It is enough if they drive us to the store where the pretend horse is and have lots of coins ready.

If they take us for walks they should slow down past pretty leaves or caterpillars. They should never say "hurry up". Usually they are fat but not too fat to tie your shoes. They can take their teeth and gums off sometimes.

It is better if they don't play cards except with us. They don't have to be smart, only answer questions like: "How come we can't see God?" and "Where does the wind come from?"

They don't talk baby talk like visitors do because it is hard to understand. When they read to us they don't skip or mind if it's the same story again. Everybody should try to have one especially if they don't have television because grandmothers are the only grown-ups who have time.

Source unknown

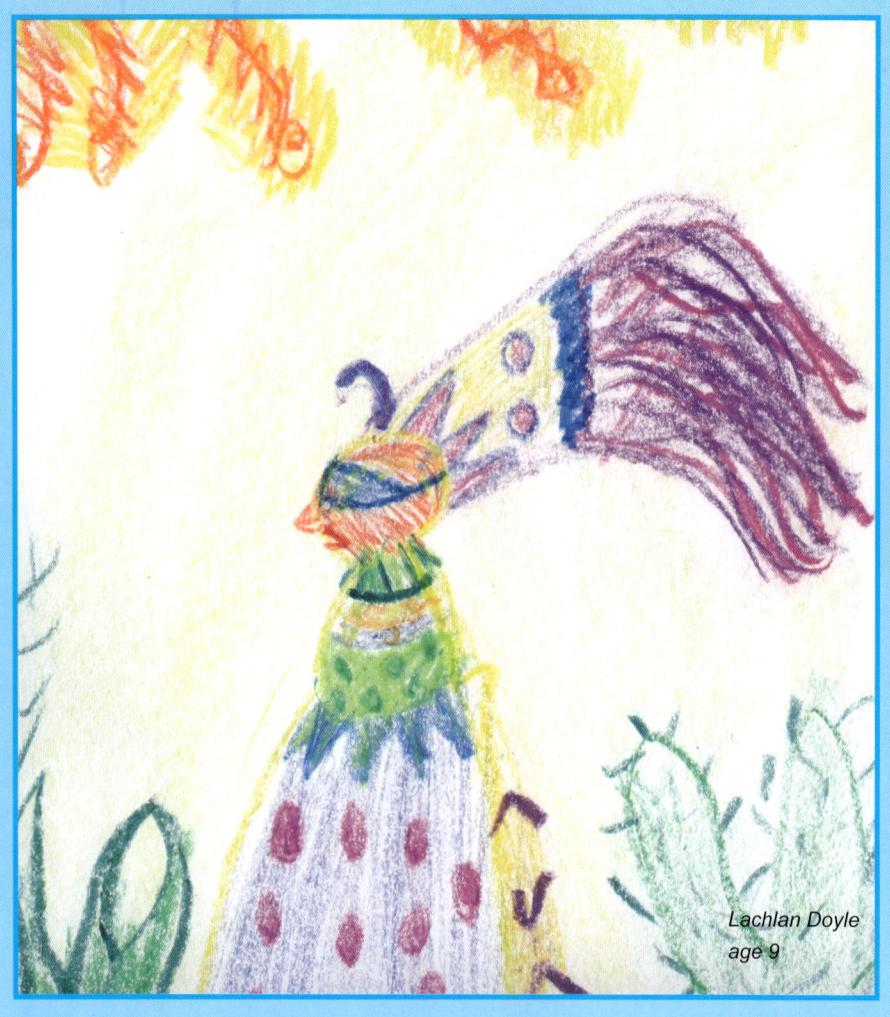

Lachlan Doyle
age 9

⭐ **Riddle**

How does a penguin build his home

⭐ **Answer**

Igloos it together!

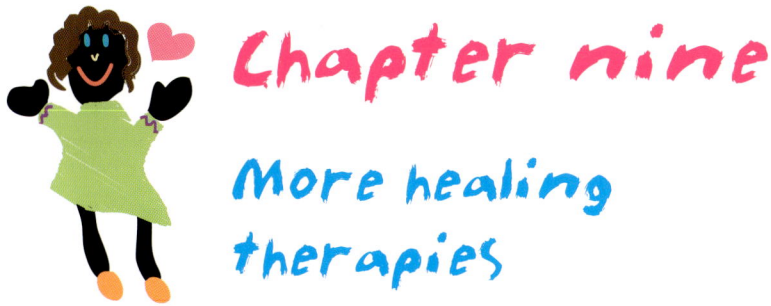

Chapter nine

More healing therapies

There are an enormous range of complementary therapy modalities available today and in this chapter I give you a brief outline of a few of my favourites, all of which are which are safe and easy for you to use at home.

Flower Remedies

Flower Essences are vibrational remedies that work on the emotional causes behind physical ailments and imbalances. They are not aromatic, but are like a homoeopathic medicine that is taken under the tongue, rubbed onto a pulse point or mixed into a hot or cold drink. The usual dosage is seven drops twice daily or as required for acute conditions. Flower remedies were originally researched and produced by Edward Bach in England. Nowadays, most countries produce their own remedies, and as a Naturopath I believe that the remedies made in your own country are most likely to be more relevant and effective.

Australian Bush Flower Essences

There are more than sixty Australian Bush Flower Essences available. These are the ones I use most frequently with children.

★ **Emergency Essence** – Helps with distress, panic and fears. It is a great essence to use after physical or emotional trauma for example, after a fall or having a nightmare.

★ **Adol Essence** – Helps with the emotional pressures and the mood changes that teenagers experience.

★ **Cognis Essence** – Gives focus and clarity when studying, speaking or reading. Assists with problem solving and accessing stored information.

★ **Confid Essence** – Brings out positive qualities of self-esteem and confidence.

★ **Relationship Essence** – Enhances communication and the ability to express feelings. Breaks negative family conditioning and enhances parent-child bonding, releasing resentment, emotional pain and turmoil.

★ **Space Clearing Essence** – Creates harmonious environments by helping to release negative emotional, physical and spiritual energy. Great for clearing tense situations and environments, and restoring balance.

Bach Flower Remedies

While the Australian Bush Flowers obviously come from Australia, the Bach remedies come from England. There are thirty-eight basic Bach remedies which have been available since early in the last century. Bach flower remedies are very popular in the northern hemisphere, and the most popular remedy is the Rescue Remedy.

★ **Rescue Remedy** — For the 'too hards'. Like the Australian Bush Flower Emergency Essences, it is commonly used for panic, anxiety and fears. Four drops are taken under the tongue or massaged onto a pulse point.

Herbal Medicine

For centuries herbs have been valued for their incredible versatility as medicines, perfumes, foods, in religious ceremonies and as simple teas; they are the oldest form of medicine on Earth and are still used as the primary form of medicine by more than 70 per cent of the world's population.

Herbs are in fact the traditional medicine of all cultures and are based on observation and experience passed down from generation to generation for thousands of years. There is an enormous body of scientific research which validates the efficacy of herbs. Herbs are the forerunners of modern pharmaceutical medicines and in fact many drugs are based on compounds found in plants. Aspirin, for example, comes from the salicylates found in Willow Bark, and heart drugs are still extracted from the Foxglove, more than two hundred years after their discovery.

While the skilled medical herbalist will conduct a consultation to assess the problem in terms of diet, lifestyle, emotional factors and other body relationships, and combine the therapeutic properties of herbs to suit the client's individual needs, even the simplest of herbal teas are able to energise, relax, restore, revitalise and assist in improving metabolic functioning. Of course, it's not just the therapeutic properties of the herbs that make you feel better; the very art of tea drinking can be beneficial as well.

Taking time and care in the preparation and serving of tea reflects a less hurried approach to life than the instant tea or coffee break that we have become more used to. The whole idea of preparing herbal tea, with its rich aromas and colours and the ritual of sitting and drinking with friends, automatically reduces our stress levels.

How to Prepare Your Herbal Teas

★ Infusions

To brew herbal tea, add one heaped teaspoon of dried herb per cup of water. Boil the water for half a minute or so and pour over the herb in a cup or teapot and allow it to steep. If the herb is made of plant leaves, brew for approximately two to three minutes. If it is made from flowers, steep a little longer (around five minutes) and if it is made from the bark, roots, seeds or fruit allow up to ten minutes in order to get maximum flavour and to extract all the nutritive minerals.

★ Decoction

Decoctions are primarily used for hard or woody plant materials such as roots, rhizomes, barks and seeds. Decoction is a form of simmering; the plant material should be crushed, cut, broken or otherwise rendered into small pieces before simmering. The method consists of placing one heaped teaspoonful of herbs per cup of cold water into a saucepan, bringing it to the boil and simmering for ten to fifteen minutes (or longer if the roots are very hard). During the entire process, the saucepan should be kept covered. Strain the brew before drinking.

How to Store Your Herb Teas

It is important to keep your herbs in airtight jars to retain their potency and flavour. If stored in clear glass jars, keep them in the dark, as light may diminish the herbs' potency. Remember that you are not the only one that enjoys the flavour and benefits of herbal teas – in hot weather weevils and other little bugs become unwelcome users of your tea, especially if your herbs are not kept in an airtight container. When stored carefully, herbs can remain fresh and potent for more than a year.

There are many herbs that are beneficial for children. The ones I most frequently recommend are:

★ **Chamomile tea** – This is best-known for the carminative and anti-inflammatory actions it has on all body systems.

★ **Lavender tea** – Like the essential oil, it is strengthening on the nervous system, soothing for skin conditions and promotes and assists relaxation and sleep.

★ **Fennel and Dill Seeds** – I particularly like this as a children's stomach and digestive system remedy for relieving flatulence and colic.

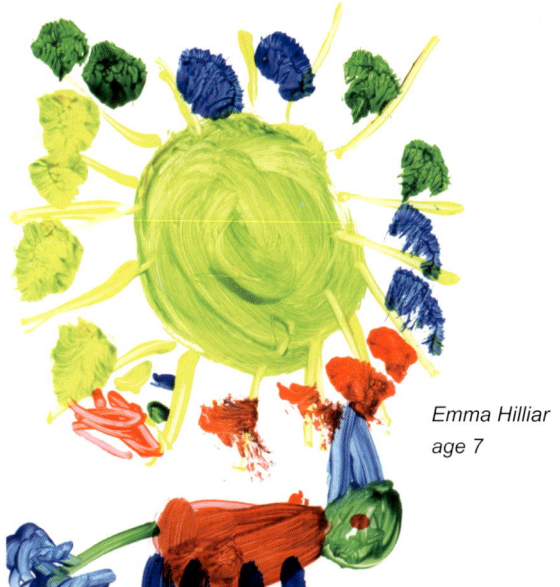

Emma Hilliar
age 7

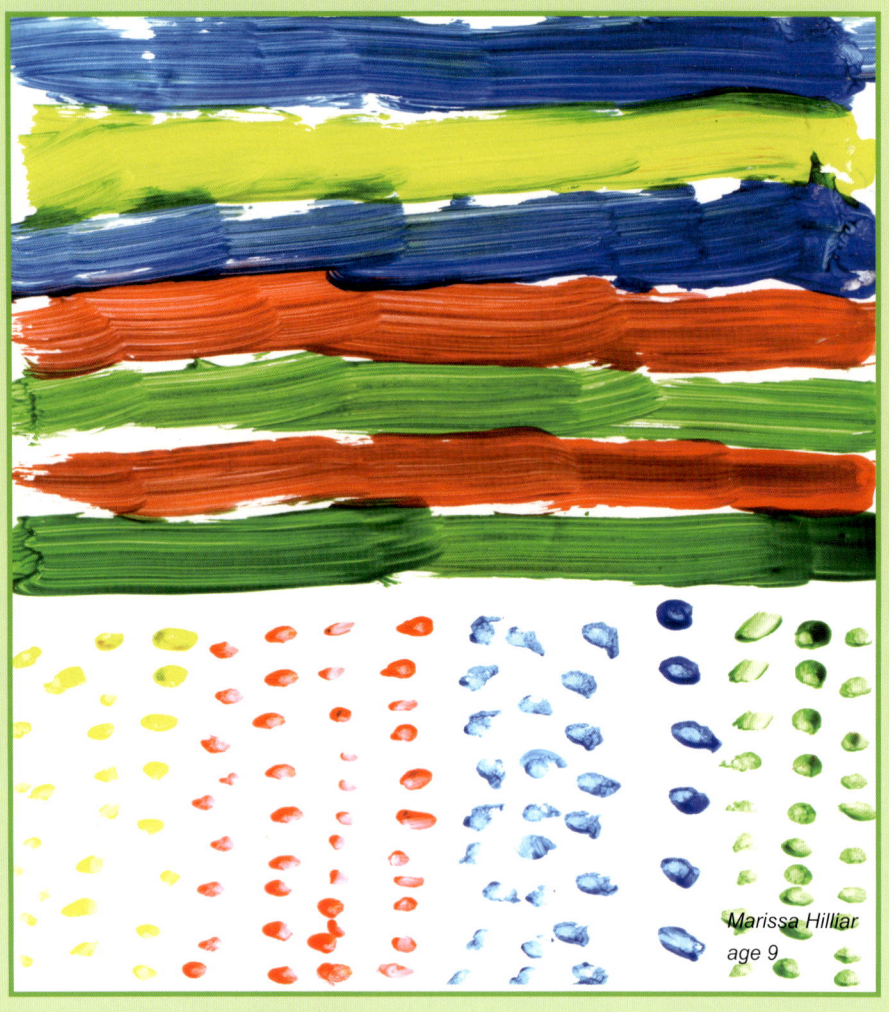

Marissa Hilliar
age 9

⭐ We can usually deflect tantrums by offering a few different choices. One particular day **Miss 3 ½** says "Mummy I don't like those choices, can you give me a few more!" ⭐

Michelle Reinhardt
Melbourne, Victoria

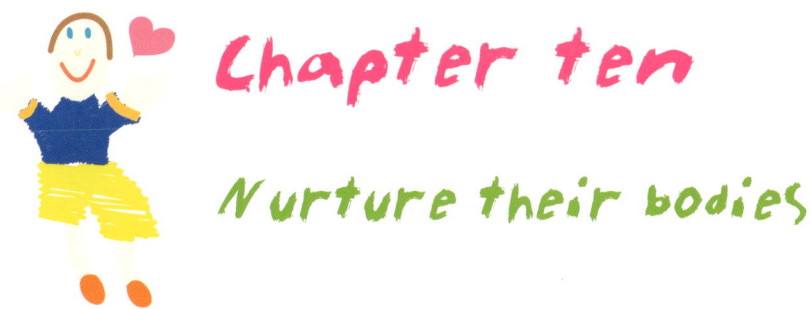

Chapter ten

Nurture their bodies

Massage has been around forever, it has always been part of healing the sick and comforting the distressed. Physically, massage improves blood circulation and lymphatic drainage, relaxes the nervous system and relieves aches, pains and muscle stiffness. Emotionally, it reduces stress and imparts a feeling of general wellbeing.

Giving a massage

Prior to beginning the massage, think happy thoughts -- the person you are massaging (whether big or small) will feel your energy through your hands. If you don't want to give a massage, don't. When you are ready, take a few deep breaths and make sure that you are completely relaxed and prepared to spend some quality time with your child.

Massage works through the empathy between the person giving the massage and the person receiving it. When giving a massage, tune into the needs of your child, concentrating on what you are feeling with your hands while listening and watching their reactions. If the intention is to give a relaxing massage, talk as little as possible. If you are simply giving a general massage after a bath, then speak pleasant, nurturing words to your child. If you are massaging an older child ask him or her to close their eyes and let their body go limp or heavy. Ask them to concentrate on their breathing or to visualise their favourite place that makes them feel relaxed.

Create a peaceful environment

★ Always massage in a warm environment, the temperature of any person being massaged, and in particular a child, may drop quite dramatically when undressed, so keep a spare towel and their clothes close by for when you have finished. Always drape a towel over the areas of the body you are not massaging, it is not just for warmth but also for that feeling of security. Take care if massaging a baby, as freshly massaged infants can be particularly slippery.

★ Avoid harsh lights that may be too bright for the child to look into while lying down. Create an environment that is soothing and nurturing. A room which is dimly lit or filled with gentle sunlight is best. Place some relaxing essential oils such as Lavender, Rosewood, Mandarin and Tangerine into a vaporiser to fragrance the room.

★ Find the position that is most comfortable for you. Try having your child on a bed, the change table or on a thick blanket or doona on the floor. You could even try laying your baby on your legs (head at your knees and bottom at your lap) while you sit leaning against a wall or lounge with your knees bent up. Remember, you need to be comfortable and take care of your posture. If massaging on a bed, kneel down rather than bending over and straining your back.

★ If you listened to some particularly soothing music while you were pregnant, you might like to play this very softly. It is reassuring for your baby to hear your voice during the massage so hum, sing or speak positive loving words.

★ If you are massaging a baby prepare a bottle for after the massage, if you are not breast-feeding.

★ Massage using long, firm strokes, with the whole hand where possible.

★ Always start at the child's legs, as this is least intrusive for them, follow your instincts and be sure that any massage on the child's tummy is done from right to left, (which will mean your left to your right).

★ Never watch the clock during massage. You will know when either you, or more importantly your child, has had enough – this is when it is time to finish.

★ Massage is beneficial to both you and your child, so take the telephone off the hook and enjoy!

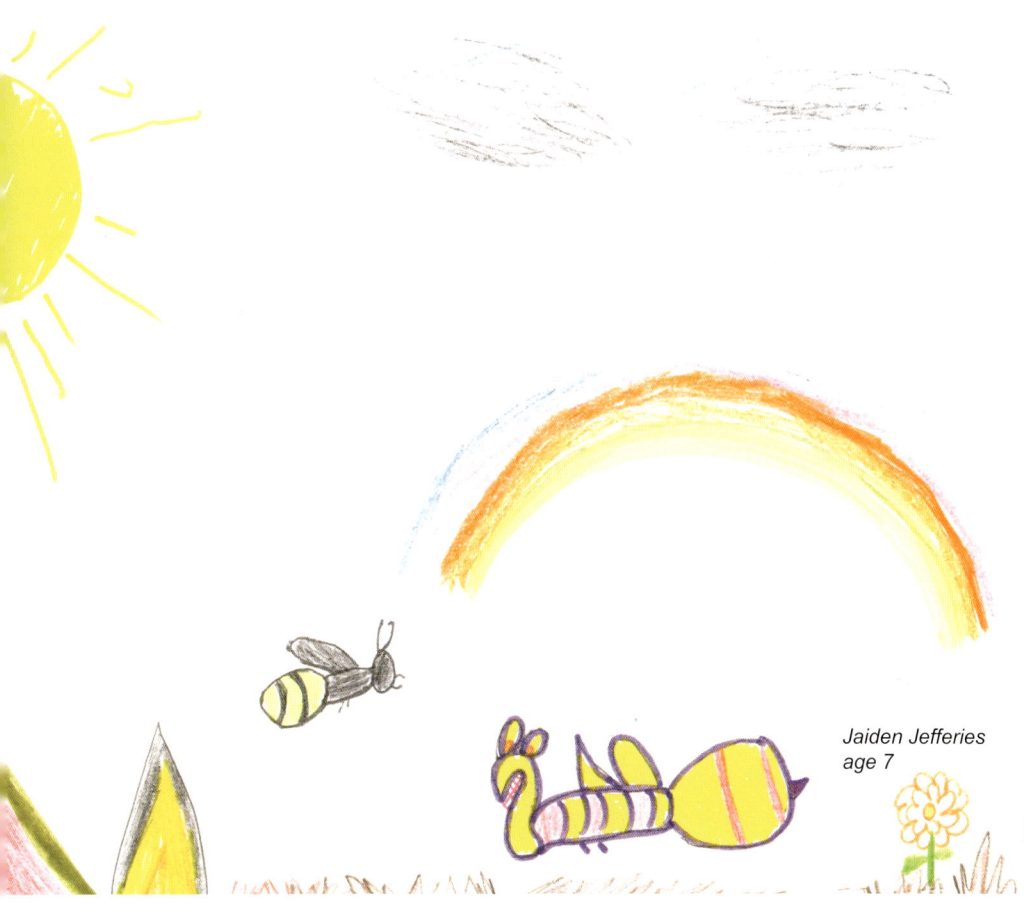

Jaiden Jefferies age 7

Points to Remember

★ Ensure that your nails are short.

★ Try to keep your hands in contact with your child throughout the massage. Constant contact assists the energy flow between you and allows your child to feel secure, to look around and take in their surroundings without having to keep checking that you are still there with them.

★ Generally, a firm but gentle touch feels good. Move more lightly over bony areas. Don't worry, you won't break your baby or child.

★ Slow movements calm while brisk movements stimulate.

★ If you forget what to do, just stroke.

★ Remember your own comfort and posture.

★ If you are going to massage an older child or partner ask them to relax and to speak as little as possible, but if something hurts or if they feel uncomfortable they should let you know.

★ Don't massage a baby straight after a feed or if they are experiencing hiccups.

★ Do not massage a newborn infant at bath time, as it can be over stimulating. If your child is four or five months or older and you want to massage at bath time, it is best to massage after the bath to allow the oil to be absorbed by the skin.

Massage Accessories

There are many massage accessories on the market, I prefer the ones made from wood. It is wonderful to get your child used to giving and receiving massage from a young age.

★ Wooden Fingers

This unique four-legged wooden massage accessory is a great device for getting into those tight spots. Just grab the top and massage with it using circular movements over the top of clothing or simply apply a little massage oil to the skin first. It is wonderful for scalp massages too.

★ Two Ball Rollers

Simply roll it up and down either side of the spine and over the shoulders to relieve stress and tension. The long handle is great as it allows you to massage your own back.

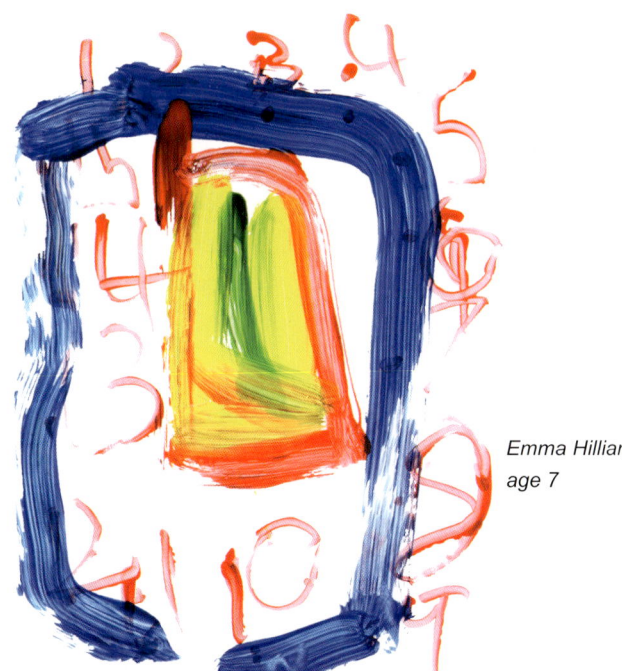

Emma Hilliar
age 7

Index

S

T

U

V

W

Y

Z

Other Books by Jennifer

★ Amazing Scents — A guide to Aromatherapy

★ 7 Steps to Sanity — How to have it all without sacrifising your health, sense of humor or sanity along the way

★ Sanity Savers — tips for work/life balance

★ The Aromatherapy Insight Cards for Intuitive Aromatherapy

★ Essential Woman — Guide to using aromatherapy for women

★ If You Want Great Skin... Throw Away Your Cosmetics

★ Network or Perish — Learn the secrets of master networkers

Visit www.jenniferjefferies.com for more information.